Mosby's
Home Health Nursing
Pocket Consultant

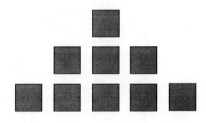

D1611693

M Mosby

St. Louis Baltimore Boston Carlsbad Chicago Naples New York
Philadelphia Portland London Madrid Mexico City Singapore
Sydney Tokyo Toronto Wiesbaden

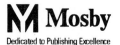 **Mosby**
Dedicated to Publishing Excellence

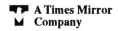 **A Times Mirror
Company**

Executive Editor: N. Darlene Como
Developmental Writer: Linda Wendling
Senior Developmental Editor: Laurie Sparks
Project Manager: Patricia Tannian
Production Editor:Barbara Jeanne Wilson
Manufacturing Manager: Theresa Fuchs
Cover Design: Gail Morey Hudson
Design and Layout: Ken Wendling

Printed in the United States of America
Composition by Wordbench
Printing/binding by R.R. Donnelly and Sons Company

Mosby–Year Book, Inc.
11830 Westline Industrial Drive
St. Louis, MO 63146

International Standard Book Number 0-8151-6125-5

93 94 95 96 97   9 8 7 6 5 4 3 2 1

Preface

As health care providers and payors looks for ways to cut health care costs, hospital stays continue to grow shorter than ever before. New mothers are routinely sent home within 24 hours of giving birth, minor surgery is frequently performed on an outpatient basis, and even clients experiencing major surgery are discharged within a few days to continue their recovery at home. As a result, there is an everincreasing need for followup nursing care at home. Procedures such as IV therapy and wound care, once the exclusive province of hospitals, are now routinely performed in the home. Home health nurses must be prepared to deal with a wide range of conditions and problems. While they can often anticipate and plan for their clients' needs in advance, they sometimes encounter unexpected problems and must be able to deal with them.

While many of the same nursing procedures are carried out in hospitals and in clients' homes, the manner in which care is provided in the home often differs significantly. It may be necessary to significantly modify how a procedure is performed and improvise equipment which is not available. Because the nurse is in the home only for a short time, clients and their families must often take an active role in providing care. Thus, educating the client and family or other caregiver is an extremely important component of home care.

Mosby's Home Health Nursing Pocket Consultant was created to address the concerns of home health nurses. It covers the entire range of home health care and addresses the diversity of problems a home health nurse is likely to see on any given day. Compact in size, it fits easily into the nurse's bag and may be taken into the home to consult as needed. At the same time, the spiral binding allows it to lay flat when opened while the wraparound flap may serve as a builtin bookmark. Information is presented concisely, in lists and tables wherever possible, to allow for quick reference. The book is divided into seven major parts. The first part, Home Health Nursing Overview, discusses the various roles of the home health nurse, case management, documentation, and thirdparty reimbursement. The second part, The Home Visit, demonstrates the steps involved in making a home visit. Important aspects of the home visit, including principles of education and communication and clients' rights, are discussed here. The third major part, Assessment, includes assessment guides for all major body systems, as well as psychosocial, functional, economic, and family assessments. Additional assessment tools are included to assist the nurse in evaluating the home environment, the client's ability to perform activities of daily living, and the client's mental status.

In the fourth major part, general considerations common to all home health clients are discussed. These include topics such as nutrition, maintaining mobility, medication administration, and infection control. The fifth part, Care of Special Patients, is devoted to the specific conditions most commonly seen in the home, including maternal and newborn care, wound care, diabetes mellitus, respiratory disorders, AIDS, stroke, chronic renal failure, Alzheimer's disease, musculoskeletal disorders, and clients needing assistance with pain control. The book concludes with appendixes which provide useful information such as brief descriptions of the various personnel involved in home care, abbreviations, guidelines for home medical equipment, Spanish-English translations for commonly used health care words and phrases, and a list of resources for additional information.

As a growing field, home health nursing is experiencing many changes. It is our hope that this reference will help the nurse adjust to these changes and provide the best possible quality care in the home.

Table of Contents

Home Health Nursing Overview

The Home Visit

Assessment

General Considerations in Caring for Clients at Home

References

Index

Home Health Nursing Overview

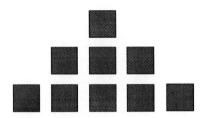

Home Health Nursing Roles

In the past several years, the provision of nursing care in the home has increased at a rate that can only be described as explosive. As the use of diagnosis-related groups (DRGs) for third-party payment has led to shortened hospital stays, clients' needs for follow-up care at home has increased. At the same time, the availability of equipment for delivering high-tech interventions in the home allows more clients to be treated in the home setting, including procedures such as renal dialysis, phototherapy, intravenous administration of antibiotics, and chemotherapy, ventilation, cardiac monitoring, and fibrillation (Redman, 1993). A final trend causing increased demand for home care services is a growing elderly population, including an increased number of frail elderly (Twardon, Gartner, & Cherry, 1993).

Home health nursing is a synthesis of community health nursing and selected technical skills from other specialty nursing practices. The American Nurses Association (ANA) asserts that "the practice of home health nursing is focused predominantly on the care of individuals, in collaboration with the family and designated caregivers" (ANA, 1992). Health care services provided in the home can range from dressing changes or insulin injections to intravenous antibiotics or dialysis. The criteria for financial coverage by providers include the following:

- The client must be homebound.
- The client must require the services of a skilled registered professional nurse or physical therapist on an intermittent basis.
- The services must be ordered by a physician.

These homebound criteria are further defined by each financially responsible party. They generally stipulate that the client be physically unable to leave the home and require the use of an ambulance or transportation agency to go to follow-up medical appointments or treatments. There are usually no exceptions to this rule. Payment for services is outlined by Medicare, Medicaid, or commercial insurance plans. Some of these guidelines will be covered later in the section on "Third-Party Reimbursement Guidelines."

The legal and professional responsibilities assumed by the home health agency include coordinating care from acceptance through discharge, providing thorough documentation for reimbursement and legal protection, and ensuring proper termination of services. The American Nurses Association states that "the goal of care (in the home) is to initiate, manage, and evaluate the resources needed to promote the client's optimal level of well-being" (Detlefs & Meyers, 1991).

Responsibilities of the Home Health Nurse

The home health nurse is responsible for implementing and evaluating the ordered plan of care. Assigning one nurse to a client helps ensure the quality of care by providing a mechanism for consistent rapport and communication with the client and caregivers.

This is not to say that additional nursing staff is not also involved in the care of that client. In fact, involving another nurse, particularly with long-term clients maintained at home, can be very helpful. In some home health agencies, a nurse specialist consults with the client and primary nurse on complex problems needing assessment and intervention. Such a process can help ensure safe, effective, quality care.

Visits made by the home health nurse are based on client needs. Naturally, the ultimate goal is successful management of health care needs at home, with clients maintaining as much control as possible over their own care. Certain universal factors that influence health care management within the client's environment include the following (Rice, 1992):

- Age-related and cultural factors
- Psychobiological factors (mental, emotional, spiritual, and physiological needs)
- Specific nature of disease and its manifestation
- Socioeconomic and environmental factors

The ANA associates the following responsibilities of care with the home health nursing profession*:

- Holistic initial and periodic assessment of the client's and caregiver's physical and financial resources to develop and support the nursing care plan
- Identification and coordination of appropriate community resources
- Qualitative and quantitative evaluation of client responses to care; monitoring of parameters of care according to the nursing care plan
- Education of clients, families, and caregivers to promote

*A Statement on the Scope of Home Health Nursing Practice, Washington, DC, 1992, American Nurses Association.

self-care activities
- Health-promotion teaching to improve the quality of life, maintain health, and minimize disability
- Advocacy through activities that inform, support, and affirm the client and family's self-determination
- Continuity of care through discharge planning, care management, and advocacy
- Application of appropriate multidisciplinary knowledge
- Recognition of developmental and biopsychosocial changes in clients and caregivers
- Use of appropriate state Nurse Practice Acts to guide nursing practice
- Technical and instrumental care
- Monitoring and support of caregiver participation

Ensuring Quality in Home Health Care

Three factors can be used to contribute to ensuring the quality of home health care within a given agency, as well as within the larger nursing community. These are accreditation, continuous quality improvement (CQI) programs, and certification.

Accreditation

Both the Joint Commission on Accreditation of Healthcare Organizations (JCAHO) and the Community Health Accreditation Program (CHAP) accredit home care programs of all types. If the program is accredited, this information and responsibilities regarding the standards and operational guidelines should be a part of every nurse's orientation.

Continuous Quality Improvement (CQI)

Orientation and accreditation are only two factors that contribute to quality in home care. Home health agencies also design and implement continuous quality improvement (CQI) programs that meet the agency's unique clinical focus. Home health agencies traditionally track the following kinds of information:
- Readmission to hospitals within 31 days
- Complaint logs
- Infection surveillance and rates
- Clinically focused studies
- 488 requests (the Medicare I Regional Home Health Intermediary [RHHI] form that requests additional, specific clinical information)

- Other aspects of home health agency operations that have an impact on care

Certification

Specialty certification is another way to help maintain and monitor quality, by ensuring that nurses in home care know and practice within standard quality parameters. The educational preparation, the clinical background, and the knowledge and experience of home care nurses can be another measure of quality. This can include the orientation process, the completed proficiency skills checklist, and the experience the nurses bring to the bedside in the home. Certification in home care is being offered by the American Nurses' Credentialing Center (Marrelli, 1994).

Qualifications of the Home Health Nurse

Home health nurses may function as either generalists or specialists. The skills required and responsibilities of each role are listed below.*

Generalist Role

- Exercise advanced assessment skills for in-depth initial and ongoing assessments for plan of care, frequency of visits, client referrals, and discharge.
- Use effective communication skills to link client, family, physician, and agency separated by distance. Accommodate culture/language barriers.
- Make independent decisions about clients' needs without the on-site support of the institutional setting; know when to proceed and when to confer.
- Demonstrate flexibility and creative problem solving in adjusting to frequently changing home and community environments; accept people's unique and chosen lifestyles and associated effects these lifestyles have on their health; bend to meet client needs and goals; improvise supplies, equipment, or therapies.
- Set up daily and weekly schedules, adding clients as requested; initiate changes in plan of care and frequency as needed; orient oneself to new settings.
- Demonstrate knowledge of the basics of home care. For

*Marrelli TM: *Handbook of home health standards and documentation guidelines for reimbursement, ed. 2,* St. Louis, 1994, Mosby-Year Book, Inc.

Medicare-certified home health agencies, know:

- The Medicare Conditions of Participation
- The HHA Health Insurance Manual (HIM-11) provisions about home care coverage
- The HIM-11 steps for correct completion of the 485 series forms
- Pay attention to detail in addressing complex client needs; provide extensive documentation.
- Have a reliable car and good driving skills, along with a willingness to drive—even in inclement weather! A good sense of direction (or a map!) is important.
- Assume complete responsibility by providing true primary care or case management, from the initial nursing assessment visit through the identification and use of appropriate nursing diagnoses. Communicate closely with the case manager and the financial providing agency.
- Possess the ability to be both specialist and generalist. Clients are of all age groups; diagnoses and care needs vary from day to day.
- Show a desire to continue learning; many new and changing technologies are being used in the home setting.
- Genuinely appreciate people, providing positive interaction and empathy for people who are in the midst of crises.
- Balance client and agency demands, recognizing that clinical and administrative demands are equally important, but in different ways.
- Keep a kind sense of humor; this can help clients and their families get through the rough times.

Specialist Role

In addition to performing all the functions of a generalist, the specialist possesses substantial clinical experience with individuals, families, and groups: expertise in the process of caseload management and consultation, and proficiency in planning, implementing, and evaluating programs, resources, services, and research for health care delivery to complex clients. The specialist in home health nursing is prepared at the graduate level. All professional nurses practicing as clinical nurse specialists in home health possess advanced nursing knowledge and skills to carry out the following responsibilities*:

---

*Marrelli TM: *Handbook of home health standards and documentation guidelines for reimbursement, ed. 2,* St. Louis, 1994, Mosby-Year Book, Inc.

- Provide consultation to the generalist who is participating in the delivery of care to high-risk home health clients.
- Design, monitor, and evaluate the continuous quality improvement process and risk management components of the clinical program.
- Identify and design research projects based on data generated from the continuous quality improvement program and clinical observations.
- Serve as a resource to the nurse generalist in the identification and evaluation of research findings for application to home health nursing practice.
- Educate the nurse generalists and health team members about technical, cognitive, and clinical developments emerging for care of the home health client.
- Perform direct care and documentation for select clients and caregivers who require specialist expertise.
- Manage and evaluate the care delivered by caregivers to prevent the recurrence of the health care deficit in complex cases.
- Design, monitor, and evaluate the caseload management system so that case mix and care demands of clients are met in an optimal manner.
- Monitor and evaluate trends and patterns of reimbursement for home health.
- Participate in developing and evaluating agency policy and procedures to promote continuity of care from preadmission to post-discharge activities.
- Facilitate a multidisciplinary and interorganizational plan of service when barriers to access and utilization are detected.
- Consult with staff and clients on ethical issues related to treatment and self-determinism.

The Home Health Nurse's Orientation

The following list addresses some of the information that an orientation should include*:
- Regulatory concerns
- Review of the state's nurse practice acts
- Occupational Safety and Health Administration (OSHA) requirements including:

*Marrelli TM: *Handbook of home health standards and documentation guidelines for reimbursement, ed. 2,* St. Louis, 1994, Mosby-Year Book, Inc.

- Hepatitis B virus vaccination
- The home health agency-related policies and supplies for bloodborne pathogens
- Universal precautions supplies, and related disposal of supplies
- Recordkeeping activities
- Medicare Conditions of Participation
- HIM-11, Revision 222, the coverage of service section
- Medicare and other insurance/provider coverage and documentation requirements
- Agency administrative issues
- Schedule of home care staff meetings
- Overview of the home health agency's medical records, documentation system, and required forms, plus orientation to automated clinical documentation system, where applicable
- Administrative details and processes
- Equipment and supply acquisition
- Benefits, employee handbook, mileage, on-call process and pay, lab pickup schedules, and other miscellaneous information unique to the program; for example:
  - Intraagency collaboration
  - Community resources
  - Safety
  - Travel
- Agency client care concerns
- Philosophy of care and scope of services
- Home health agency's orientation and clinical policy and procedure manual(s)
- Discussion of ethical questions
- Peer observations in joint field visits
- Introduction to clinical nurse specialists
- Introduction to ancillary services
- Home improvisation
- Guidelines for home visits
- Opportunity to "buddy" with an experienced home health agency nurse
- Continuous quality improvement (CQI) processes

Ethical Considerations
for the Home Health Nurse

In recent years, advances in technology have shaped concerns about ethics in health care, particularly regarding the allocation of health care resources and the use of advanced technology to extend a client's life. Home health nurses must grapple with principles of autonomy, beneficence, nonmaleficence, justice, confidentiality, and truth telling.

Premature discharge of clients based on expired or diminished reimbursement sources can influence the decision to provide home care. Clients who are underserved and families who are unable to successfully meet the demands of care can pose difficult problems for the health care organization and nurse. Clients, families, and caregivers may demand services that are not required or covered by insurance sources, reject reasonable and beneficial treatment and planning activities, refuse to improve environmental conditions essential to the plan of care, or avoid reporting abuse or neglect. Many situations in home health involve the autonomous concerns of different parties—the agency and nurse provider, the client, the family caregivers, the community, and the third-party payer.

The nature of home health care demands the mediation of values, obligations, and interests of formal and informal care providers. Home health care promotes active participation of the client and family in caregiving activities. Collaboration with the family and client on visit time and duration can reduce the disruption of the home routines. The home environment must be respected in a different manner from an institutional environment. An awareness of this issue promotes mutual acceptance of the professional visit (Marrelli, 1994).

Case Management

Case management is the process of planning, organizing, coordinating, and monitoring services and resources needed to respond to an individual's health care needs. It supports the effective use of health care and social services. Its goals are to provide quality health care, decrease fragmentation, enhance the client's quality of life, and contain costs (Stanhope, 1992). Table 1 compares case management and the nursing process.

Table 1   The Nursing Process and Case Management

Nursing Process	Case Management Process	Activities Involved
Assessment	Casefinding and Assessment	Develop networks with target population; seek referrals; apply screening tools according to program goals and objectives; apply comprehensive assessment methods; perform interdisciplinary, family, and client conferences
Diagnosis	Problem Identification	Determine conclusion based on assessment; use interdisciplinary team

(Continued)

Table 1   The Nursing Process and Case Management (cont'd)

Nursing Process	Case Management Process	Activities Involved
Planning	Problem Prioritizing	Validate and prioritize problems with all participants; develop activities, time-frames, and options; gain client's consent to implement plan; have client choose options
Implementation	Client Advocacy	Contact providers; negotiate services and prices; coordinate service delivery; monitor for changes in client or service status
Evaluation	Reassessment	Examine outcomes against goals; examine needs against service; examine costs; examine satisfaction of client, providers, and case manager

Stanhope M and Lancaster J: *Community health nursing: Process and practice for promoting health, ed. 3*, St. Louis, 1992, Mosby-Year Book, Inc.

Roles and Characteristics

As direct care needs of clients become increasingly complex, the intensity and duration of activities required to attend to case management alone increases. Case management responsibilities include the following duties*:

Client evaluation	Treatment plan coordination
Family evaluation	Monitoring client progress
Provider evaluation	Ancillary service coordination
Communication facilitation	Cost-benefit analysis assistance

To be an efficient case manager, the home health nurse should be able to do all of the following:

- Understand and evaluate specific diagnoses (utilizing significant clinical credentials and experience).
- Understand and explain in simple terms technical medical language and terminology.
- Maintain an appropriate balance between assertiveness and diplomacy with people at all levels.
- Objectively assess situations to determine the appropriateness of case management.
- Be aware of available resources and the strengths and weaknesses of each.
- Be familiar with employee benefits, eligibility, and insurance concerns.
- Act as advocate for client and payer in models relying on third-party payment.
- Act as a counselor to clients, providing support, understanding, information, and intervention.

*Stanhope M and Lancaster J: *Community health nursing: Process and practice for promoting health, ed. 3*, St. Louis, 1992, Mosby-Year Book, Inc.

Frequency and Length of Service Considerations

Early discharge and shorter lengths of stay in acute care facilities have resulted in a greater number of high acuity home care clients. These clients require services necessitating expanded skills and increased knowledge on the part of the home health nurse. The increasing complexity of client needs is demonstrated in the changing case mix of the home health nurse's case load. The introduction of diagnosis-related groups (DRGs) and other prospective payment systems in inpatient settings has increased the scrutiny of admission, frequency, and duration of home health services.

In addition, most health care analysts, payers, and consumers of health care realize that forms of prospective payment systems, such as the Medicare hospice benefit, will continue to expand to other areas of health care, including home health care.

The frequency of visits and the length of service are usually based on the professional nurse's assessment and ongoing evaluation of the client's clinical status, as well as on his or her biopsychosocial and unique family system needs. All visits require orders by the physician, and the nurse must maintain compliance with the Medicare Conditions of Participation, state licensure, surveyor directives, and other regulations or laws. This is done in part through ongoing meetings with the home health care manager to determine clients' unique frequency and duration needs (Marrelli, 1994).

Defining Frequency and Duration

In the text addressing the completion of element 21 on the HCFA form 485, the HIM-11 manual states, "Frequency denotes the number of visits per discipline to be rendered, stated in days, weeks, or months. Duration identifies the length of time the services are to be rendered and may be expressed in days, weeks, or months." For this discussion, duration, usually referred to as 60 to 62 days, is the length of stay (LOS) for which the client is projected to need home care services in order to safely and effectively meet the client's unique medical and other needs.

Naturally, the most important considerations to keep in mind when determining frequency and duration are recognized medical or nursing practice standards. At the same time, realistically and operationally, other factors are also important to scheduling and frequency decisions. These include the following (Marrelli, 1994):

- Staffing trends
- Standards of practice
- Geographic location of client's, family, and referral support systems
- Availability of qualified staff for clients with particular conditions or problems

Client-Related Considerations

The following is a list of the most common client-related considerations that are evaluated by the nurse as plans are formulated and care is begun. It is not all-inclusive; other considerations may be as varied as the individual nurse's client caseload. In addition, many of these factors are interrelated.

Absence of caregiver
Activities of daily living (ADL) limitations
Adaptive or assistive devices
Affect (e.g., depression)
Behavioral or mental disorders
Caregiver support
Chemical or drug problems (e.g., alcoholism)
Chronic illness(es)
Cognitive function
Communication
Compliance/noncompliance
Disabilities
Discharge plan
Drug interactions
Educational level/barriers
Environment
Fatigue
Fire safety
Functional limitations
Goals/expected outcomes
Handicaps
History
Home medical equipment
Home setting
Independence
Instrumental activities of daily living (IADL)

Knowledge of emergency procedures
Language
Loneliness
Loss of significant other(s)
Medical equipment or supply needs
Medications
Mobility
Motivation
Nursing assessment and reassessment findings
Nursing diagnoses
Nutritional status
Orthotic needs
Other considerations based on client's/family's unique needs
Pain
Parenting
Pathology
Physical assessment findings
Polypharmacy
Probability of further complications
Prognosis
Psychopathology
Reason for prior hospilalization, for referral to home
    care/hospice
Rehabilitative needs
Resources (e.g., financial, human, and other)
Risk factors
Safety
Self-care status
Skin integrity
Social factors
Social supports
Socioeconomic condition
Stability
Swallowing
Voice

Home health nurses, managers, and administrators must articulate to a case manager or third-party payer the objective rationale and plan for projected visits. Nurses must be able to communicate objectively the skills used during every visit and explain why those visits may vary, even though clients may have the same general diagnoses or problems.

Research-based practice guidelines, outcome measures, and standards of care are important because of the increased emphasis on cost-effective, high-quality care. These practice parameters can help home care nurses determine client frequency and length of service.

Some home health agencies have developed their own standardized care plans based on North American Nursing Diagnosis Association (NANDA) nursing diagnoses and the nurses' experience with particular client problems. Other home health agencies have developed or purchased automated systems that help them track and define objective findings, demonstrate goal achievement, and discharge based on outcome criteria. Nurses in practice are aware of this ongoing concern regarding provision of adequate client care in a climate of tighter reimbursement, more limited resources, and frequent ethical dilemmas, along with an emphasis on both quality and effectiveness. Table 2 shows suggested schedules for the home health nurse (RN), based on varying discharge goals. This cost/quality equation must balance out in order to maintain client satisfaction, success productivity, and viability of the health care organization as well as the nurse's satisfaction in the ability to meet client need (Marrelli, 1994).

Table 2   Suggested Schedules for Home Visits

Nurse (RN)
  Discharge Goals:

1 Month	1 1/2 - 2 Months	2 - 3 Months
x1-2/wk: 1-2 wk	x3/wk: 1-2 wk	x3/wk: 1-2 wk
q2wk: x1-2	x2/wk: 1 wk	x2/wk: 2-3 wk
	x1/wk: 1-2 wk	x1/wk: 2-4 wk
	q2wk: x1-2	q2wk: x1

Physical Therapist (PT)
  Discharge of 1 - 2 months

x3/wk: 2-3 wk	x2-3 wk: 6-8 wk
x2/wk: 1-2 wk	or
x1/wk: 1-2 wk	x1-2 wk: 2-3 wk

(Continued)

Table 2   Suggested Schedules for Home Visits (cont'd)

Occupational Therapist (OT)

---

x1 - 2/wk: 2 - 3 wk
x1/wk: 3 - 4 wk
x2 - 3/wk: 6 - 8 wk

Social Worker (MSW)

---

2 - 3 visits; repeat and document as needed for additional monthly visits.

Speech Therapist (ST)

---

x3/wk: 3 - 4 wk
x2 - 3/wk: 3 - 4 wk
x2/wk: 2 - 3 wk

Home Health Aide (HHA)

---

x3 - 4 wk: frequency and length of visits depend on medical necessity for personal care, e.g., bed-bound, extreme weakness, severe exertional dyspnea.

Adapted from Jaffe MS and Skidmore-Roth L: *Home health nursing care plans, ed. 2*, St. Louis, 1993, Mosby-Year Book, Inc.

Third-Party Reimbursement Guidelines

The following are intended only to be used as rough guidelines for Medicare, Medicaid, CHAMPUS, and private health insurance reimbursments. In addition to these, it is important to consult the guidelines set forth in a client's specific policy*:

- Medicare benefits for health care are available to most clients who are over 65 years of age, disabled for 2 years or more, or on renal dialysis. These clients also may have supplemental private health insurance that covers expenses that Medicare does not pay; these plans vary and benefits are policy specific.
- Medicaid is a government assistance plan that differs from state to state. Coverage is reserved for a segment of the population whose economic status complies with the payment standards set by government regulations (usually 50% federal and 50% state funded).
- CHAMPUS insurance benefits and coverage are reserved for government employees eligible to receive these payments via past or present employment or service to the government.
- Private health insurance may be individually owned and paid for or part of a group policy sponsored and paid for completely or in part by the client's employer.
- Private long-term care insurance may include home care benefits following a hospitalization or long-term facility stay, or it may be for home care exclusively as a single policy or as a rider to a long-term nursing home policy.
- Requirements and benefits for government and private insurance change periodically; major areas of coverage usually include client assessment, teaching, and performing complex procedures, with hours or number of visits allowed depending on acuity and type of skilled care needed; skilled care is needed before a home health aide will be paid.
- Medicare, Medicaid, and third-party payers require documentation of homebound status and skilled care need (varies from state to state), with specific, detailed functional limitations included in the medical diagnoses; for example: "acute exacerbation of rheumatoid arthritis on (date) with inability to move from bed to chair." They also require a medical

*Adapted from Jaffe MS and Skidmore-Roth L: *Home health nursing care plans, ed. 2*, St. Louis, 1993, Mosby-Year Book, Inc.

plan of care and medical orders for home care.

- The medical diagnosis should include an appropriate adjective for a better description; for example: "uncontrolled diabetes." Give the most acute diagnosis as the principal diagnosis, and include the dates of onset.
- Care plans are initially developed by a nurse after an appropriate nursing history and assessments of client are completed, or they may be developed by a physical, occupational, or speech therapist.
- Discharge must be considered if nursing interventions are not needed for up to 3 weeks and no problems exist or recur for which Medicare benefits would apply.
- Specific nursing diagnoses that identify nursing problems, as opposed to medical diagnoses, which identify medical conditions, are required; for example:
  "Diabetes mellitus: Knowledge deficit related to subcutaneous administration of insulin."
- Goals must be written as "outcomes," which are to be achieved in a specific period of time (e.g., short-term and long-term). The examples that follow are goals for client and for nurse:
  - Client states purpose of insulin, action, dosage, time, and side effects (expected within 3 days or during second visit).
  - Teach client insulin administration (expected within 10 days or by end of fourth visit).
- Goals must reflect nursing diagnosis and specify actions expected to solve the problems stated in the diagnosis; this may vary with Medicare requirements.
- Interventions are the stated actions that the nurse, client, and family or caretaker complete to achieve the goals. Specific skilled care and teaching that relate to the diagnosis and physician orders should be delineated. A list of specific personnel performing interventions should be included with the activities in the care plan.
- Nursing diagnoses and interventions are listed in order of priority. Medicare and insurance plans do not pay for maintenance care except in the case of a private insurance plan that is specifically for long-term care, although Medicaid will sometimes pay for skilled management for short-term care.
- The review or evaluation includes dates when goals are expected to be achieved or not achieved.
- The frequency of paid visits depends on the diagnosis, the acuteness of the condition, client's or caretaker's ability to

learn, presence of a caretaker to teach, stability of client's condition, and multiple medical diagnoses. Parameters may or may not be given as a basis for the number of visits that would be acceptable. Start with a higher frequency of visits; then taper down if possible and schedule for 2 or 3 times per week. Daily visits are usually allowed only for an acute phase or teaching; however, proper documentation will allow for daily or twice-daily visits to be covered by Medicare.

- The nurse assesses need for physical therapy, but physician order is needed for this referral.
- The physical therapy, occupational therapy, and referral for social worker are ordered by the physician.
- A home health aide may be placed in the home if no one is able to perform personal care for the client; this care by an aide is allowed only if skilled care is also needed for the client for Medicare and Medicaid benefits.
- At lease two of the following skilled care interventions are necessary for Medicare payment:
  - Assessment and evaluation
  - Hands-on care and procedures
  - Teaching
- Visits should be determined by individual need and agency policy, physician orders, homebound status, insurance criteria, and the need for skilled care and intermittent care. Table 2 shows suggested schedules for the home health nurse (RN), based on varying discharge goals.

Documentation

Today, numerous third-party payers make quality and reimbursement decisions based on the care the client received as evidenced in the medical record. The professional home care nurse's entries in a client's clinical record are recognized as a significant contribution that documents the standard of care provided to a client. As the practice of nursing has become more complex, so too have the factors that influence documentation. These factors include requirements of regulatory agencies (e.g., the state health department); third-party payers (Medicare, Medicaid, and private insurance); accreditation organizations (e.g., JCAHO, CHAP); consumers of health care; and legal entities. In addition, the written clinical record is the nurse's best defense against malpractice or negligence litigation.

The clinical record is the only source of written communication, and sometimes the only source of any communication, for all team members. The team members not only contribute their unique and individual assessments of interventions and outcomes, but may also actually base their subsequent actions on the events documented by another team member.

Actual documentation should be completed as soon as possible. This includes beginning the HCFA form 485 (or other required forms) and the daily visit record or nursing notes as soon as possible (Marrelli, 1994).

Factors Contributing to More Emphasis on Nursing Documentation

Five specific areas have increased the importance of nursing and clinical documentation*:

- *The current economics of our health care system and the emphasis on utilization management.* In response to spiraling health care costs, third-party payers have increased their scrutiny and control of limited resources. Clients are released from hospitals and similar facilities "quicker and sicker." In general, the decreased length of hospital stays has increased home care clients' acuity levels. This often translates into increased

*Marrelli TM: *Handbook of home health standards and documentation guidelines for reimbursement, ed. 2,* St. Louis, 1994, Mosby-Year Book, Inc.

nursing care and other needs and is evidenced by the increase in the number of visits or hours clients are seen. At the same time, some managed-care programs are decreasing the number of home visits allowed while also limiting the client's hospital stay. This places stress on the home health nurse to continue to provide needed care and many times "negotiate" for the client so that the appropriate level of safe, effective nursing care is provided. Third-party payers often need substantiating evidence—documentation—that clearly shows skilled care was provided. The information in the clinical record is the source by which third-party payers make payment or denial decisions.

Some conditions indicating homebound status are:

- Fractures or disabilities that prevent ambulation without assistance or use of assistive aids or that prevent weight bearing or the use of arms to open doors, etc.
- Shortness of breath with slight exertion, as in chronic obstructive pulmonary disease or chronic heart failure
- Weakness as the result of surgery or illness or client being easily fatigued
- Dizziness, weakness, poor balance, or unsteady gait
- Incision, draining wound, or dressing changes
- Indwelling catheter
- Wheelchair- or bed-bound
- Sensory deficiencies such as visual or auditory impairment or aphasia
- Paraplegia, quadriplegia, hemiplegia, numbness of extremities, paresis, or impaired peripheral circulation
- Mental confusion, extreme anxiety, or paranoia
- Obesity if mobility is compromised
- Severe pain
- Inability to communicate effectively
- Unstable blood glucose levels causing weakness and dizziness

- *The emphasis on CQI in home care.* As quality initiatives in all health care settings have evolved, client outcomes are being recognized as valid indicators of care. The interdisciplinary focus on quality efforts creates an incentive for the entire health team to work together to achieve client outcomes.
- *The emphasis on standardization of care, policies, and procedures.* All clients are entitled to a certain level or standard of nursing care. As clients become more proactive consumers in their purchase of health services, client satisfaction with the care provided is key to any home health agency's reputation and ultimate survival.

- *As a legal record.* As society has become litigious, the home health nurse must be aware of state practice and other accepted standards of care. These standards necessitate keeping current and informed of the standards of professional nursing practice through affiliation with nursing specialty groups or other professional groups.
- *The emphasis on effectiveness and efficiency in all settings in health care, particularly home care.* As home health agencies and all health care settings continue to streamline their operations, administrative tasks historically performed by nurses are being reconsidered for their effectiveness. Repetition or duplication of documentation has been an area of appropriate concern to both home health nurses and their managers. Some home care programs have moved toward automation to help prevent duplication (Marrelli, 1994).

Table 3 Do's and Don'ts for Effective Documentation

Do	Don't
Write legibly or print neatly. The record must be readable. Use permanent ink.	Cross out words beyond recognition.
Describe care or interventions provided and the client's response to care.	Chart care that you did not provide.
For every entry, problem, or nursing diagnosis in the care plan, identify the time and date; sign the entry and include your title.	Leave blank spaces between entries and your signature.
Make sure the client's name is listed and correct on the visit record, daily note, or other agency form.	Leave gaps in documentation or neglect to record the client's name.

(Continued)

Table 3   Do's and Don'ts for Effective Documentation (cont'd)

Do	Don't
Write notes in consecutive and chronological order with no skipped lines or gaps. Indicate in the care plan the time-frames in which care will be provided, such as 2 to 3 times per week or less, depending on condition and insurance parameters.	Write notes in a haphazard order, skipping sections to complete later.
Write down the client's, family's, or caregiver's response to teaching or any other care intervention.	Assume that responses by the client or family are less important and "okay to skip over."
Write objectively when describing findings (e.g., behaviors).	Make assumptions, draw conclusions, or blame.
Use specific, objective observations, such as: "able to ambulate only 10 feet without fatigue" or "reddened area on right heel, 1 cm in diameter."	Inject subjective, indistinct information, such as: "general weakness" or "reddened heel."
Document client complaints or needs and their resolutions. (Remember to also discuss the complaint with your manager, who may also document it in the agency's Complaint Log and note the resolution or follow-up actions taken.)	Attempt to deal with complaints while avoiding their documentation or not reporting them to the agency.

(Continued)

Table 3   Do's and Don'ts for Effective Documentation (cont'd)

Do	Don't
Use client, family, or caregiver quotes. Be accurate, complete, and thorough. Be factual and specific.	Paraphrase important responses.
Promptly document any change and the actions taken. Write visit notes either at the client's home (if safe and appropriate) or as soon as possible after care is provided.	Rely on memory or wait "too long" to record entries.
Write out what you are saying if anything is questionable. (Avoid potentially confusing abbreviations.)	Use abbreviations except where they are clear and appear on the agency's list of approved, acceptable abbreviations.
To correct an error: (1) draw a line through the erroneous entry; (2) briefly describe the error (e.g., wrong date, spilled coffee on visit record); and (3) add your signature, date, and time.	White out or erase entries; such changes may appear to be an attempt to cover up incriminating entries.

Adapted from Marrelli TM: *Handbook of home health standards and documentation guidelines for reimbursement, ed. 2*, St. Louis, 1994, Mosby-Year Book, Inc.

A Final Checklist for Effective Documentation

In addition to the suggestions in Table 3, the following list offers several strategies for ensuring that quality and reimbursement requirements are being met*:

- At the first visit, initiate the process of claims payment.
- Read your documentation as objectively as possible to see if it reflects why the client is homebound and how or why the skills of a nurse or therapist are needed.
- Emphasize (1) why the care was initiated, (2) what the skilled nursing interventions are, (3) where the client's plan is going (client-centered goals), and (4) what the plans are for discharge (rehabilitation potential).
- The plan of care is the most important part of the home care clinical record. Even though the HCFA form 485 reads "Plan of Treatment" across the top, it is referred to as the POC. The POC must be complete and the content clear. There can be no gaps.
- Make sure your clients meet the home health agency's and insurance program's admission criteria.
- Demonstrate through your documentation that the care provided is client-centered.
- Demonstrate the nursing process in the record. Look for the nursing diagnoses, the assessment, evidence of care planning, implementation of ordered interventions and actions, movement toward client-centered goals, assessment of the client's response, and continued evaluation.
- Document goal achievement and/or progress toward goals and outcomes.
- If progress has not occurred as planned, give the reasons in the documentation. If a client is too ill for a rehabilitation service or refuses the service, is there evidence of communication with the doctor about this?
- Document evidence of "intradisciplinary" team conferences and discussions.
- The chart should show continuity of care planning goals and consistent movement toward goal achievement by all

*Adapted from Marrelli TM: *Handbook of home health standards and documentation guidelines for reimbursment, ed. 2*, St. Louis, 1994, Mosby-Year Book, Inc.

members of the health team.

- Document unstable states that require interventions such as medication or catheter changes, sterile irrigations, pulmonary physiotherapy, and others that need skilled nursing care; document response to medication and treatment changes. Make sure that skilled care matches the diagnoses and physician orders.
- Finally, the clinical documentation should demonstrate compliance with regulatory, licensure, and quality standards.

Requirements for Documentation of Supervisory Visits

Documentation done weekly should indicate that client is homebound, with specific notation of physical, mental, or emotional limitations or restrictions that would not allow leaving home. Homebound status is determined by state for Medicaid or third-party payer; Medicare allows leaving home for short periods of time if infrequent. Notes should not indicate activities done outside the home except physical or laboratory appointments, providing the frequency would not indicate the possibility of outpatient care (Jaffe & Skidmore-Roth, 1993).

- Supervision for licensed vocational nurse (LVN) or home health aide (HHA) specific to payment source, including notation about client and family expression of satisfaction with care; comprehension of care plan by LVN or HHA, support given and encouragement in ADL progression with or without assistance, and responses; continuation or withdrawal of LVN or HHA
- Assigning registered nurse, physical therapist, occupational therapist, or other professional to provide care; removal when care completed
- Summary of care plan for past 2 to 3 weeks
- Client and family responses regarding care
- Evaluation of care and needs provided by LVN or HHA
- Care plan revision if needed or restatement of the existing plan
- When to review plan, usually in 2 to 4 weeks (every 2 weeks for Medicare, every 4 weeks for Medicaid and third-party payers)
- Signature and date

The Home Visit

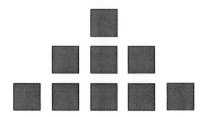

Phases and Activities of a Home Visit

For the duration of the home health services, the same nurse generally performs initial and ongoing assessment, implements and evaluates the ordered plan of care (POC), supplies documentation, acts as a liaison, and works toward discharge from home services. For each visit, such activities actually begin before the visit itself and extend beyond until a summary is written and the next visit is planned. Table 4 outlines these phases and associated activities.

Table 4   Phases and Activities of a Home Visit

Phase	Activity
I. Initiation phase	Clarify source of referral for visit
	Clarify purpose for home visit
	Share information on reason and purpose of home visit with client and family
II. Previsit phase	Initiate contact with client and family
	Establish shared perception of purpose with client and family
	Determine family's willingness for home visit
	Schedule home visit
	Review referral and/or family record
	Identify payment source

(Continued)

Table 4   Phases and Activities of a Home Visit (cont'd)

Phase	Activity
III. In-home phase	Introduction of self and professional identity
	Social interaction to establish rapport
	Establish nurse-client relationship
	Implement nursing process
IV. Termination phase	Review visit with family
	Plan for future visits
V. Postvisit phase	Record visit
	Plan for next visit

Adapted from Stanhope M and Lancaster J: *Community health nursing: Process and practice for promoting health, ed. 3,* St. Louis, 1992, Mosby-Year Book, Inc.

Therapeutic Communication

The purpose of the initial client interview is to gather data, establish rapport, and lay a foundation for trust between the client and the nurse. An expression of warmth and respect by the nurse facilitates this exchange. Give the person special attention at the beginning of the intererview by calling the client by name and using appropriate touch. The nurse must clearly state any expectations and assess the client's understanding of the communication. Therapeutic communication techniques are valuable. However, an attitude of caring is the foundation of therapeutic transaction. The nurse should be aware of actions that often block communication.

After the initial interview, a therapeutic communication process is established. Empathetic communication is a skill acquired through self-awareness and perceptive listening. These guidelines can be integrated so that the client is the focus of the verbal and the nonverbal exchange (Goodner & Skidmore-Roth, 1993).

Table 5 outlines both aids and barriers to good communication with the client.

Table 5 Aids and Barriers to Therapeutic Communication

Communication Aids	Barriers
Providing privacy	Asking persistent, probing questions
Letting the client set the pace of the exchange; giving the client time to organize thoughts	Asking one question after another or implying that you are in a hurry or preoccupied
Encouraging talk by using silence	Interrupting
Encouraging expression of feelings; awareness of anxiety cues exhibited (e.g., nervous laughing or restlessness)	Discounting client's emotional experience or "lecturing"

(Continued)

**Table 5   Aids and Barriers to
                 Therapeutic Communication (cont'd)**

Communication Aids	Barriers
Maintaining a nonjudgmental attitude	Allowing confrontation
Conducting short interviews	Letting the client get tired or bored
Asking one question at a time	Asking a barrage of unrelated questions
Asking open-ended questions and clarifying statements when necessary	Asking "yes-and-no" or leading questions that suggest an expected answer
Using positive nonverbal communication (leaning forward, maintaining eye contact, smiling, using light humor when appropriate); maintaining congruency in verbal and body language	Staring; avoiding eye contact; making faces to oneself or a peer; showing anger or anxiety, especially when these will provoke a negative reaction
Choosing clear, concise words adapted to the individual's needs (only if needed); encouraging mutual, intuitive understanding that allows client to clarify	Using phrases or slang that can be misinterpreted; using words the client does not understand or "talking down" to a client; using inappropriate cliches
Being honest; having genuine empathy	Giving false reassurance; being insincere
Saying nonverbally or verbally, "I care about you"	Offering counseling when the timing is wrong or when the client is not ready to hear what is being communicated; do not say, "I understand"

(Continued)

Table 5   Aids and Barriers to Therapeutic Communication (cont'd)

Communication Aids	Barriers
Teaching and informing only; explaining to the client how information will be used; repeating important points you want the client to remember; summarizing at the end of the conversation to focus on the important points and validate the client's understanding	Giving unwarranted advice; expressing opinions
Offering to collaborate with the client on resolving problems	Attempting to "take control" and/or solve the client's problems for him or her
Exploring ideas completely	Dropping a subject (that the client has brought up) without some resolution
Clarifying thoughts when necessary; paraphrasing statements and feelings to facilitate further talking; translating feelings into words to bring out hidden meanings	Trying to read the client's mind
Focusing on reality, especially if the client misinterprets facts or if he or she is misrepresenting the truth	"Going along" with a client's "story"; assuming the client can't be challenged or told the truth
Encouraging mutual, intuitive understanding; encouraging the client to ask for clarification if he or she does not understand what is being said	Using phrases or slang that can be misunderstood and using words that the client does not understand or inappropriate cliches

Adapted from Goodner B: *The nurse's survival guide, ed. 2*, El Paso, Tex., 1993, Skidmore-Roth Publishing.

Breaking Through Cultural Barriers to Communication

All of the strategies used to communicate with clients in general should be applied to clients from different cultures. In addition, there are several other steps you can take to ensure clear and effective communication with clients from other cultures.*

Step 1   Assess your attitudes about persons from other cultures.

- Review your personal beliefs and past experiences.
- Set aside any attitudes, values, and biases that are judgmental.

Step 2   Assess communications variables from a cultural perspective.

- Determine the client's ethnic identity, including generation in America.
- Use the client as a source of information when possible.
- Assess cultural factors that may affect your relationship with the client and respond appropriately.

Step 3   Plan care based on the communicated needs and cultural background.

- Learn as much as possible about the client's cultural customs and beliefs.
- Encourage the client to reveal cultural interpretation of health, illness, and health care.
- Be sensitive to the uniqueness of the client.
- Identify sources of discrepancy between the client's and your own conceptions of health and illness.
- Communicate at the client's level of functioning.

Step 4   Modify communication to meet cultural needs.

- Be attentive to signs of fear, anxiety, and confusion in the client. Be alert for feedback that the client is not understanding.
- Do not assume meaning is interpreted without distortion.
- Respond in a reassuring manner in keeping with the client's

*Adapted from Giger J and Davidhizar R: *Transcultural nursing, ed. 2,* St. Louis, 1995, Mosby (in press).

cultural orientation.

- Be alert to words the client seems to understand and use them frequently.
- Keep messages simple and repeat them frequently.
- Avoid using medical terms and abbreviations which the client may not understand.
- Be aware that in some cultural groups discussion with others concerning the client may offend and impede nursing process.
- Use an appropriate language dictionary. The Spanish-English equivalency chart in this book may help.

Step 5 Respect the client and his or her communicated needs.

- Use a kind and attentive approach to convey respect.
- Learn how listening is communicated in the client's culture; then use appropriate active listening techniques.
- Adopt an attitude of flexibility, respect, and interest to help bridge barriers imposed by culture.
- Be considerate of reluctance to talk when the subject involves sexual matters; be aware that in some cultures, sexual matters are not discussed freely with members of the opposite sex.

Step 6 Communicate in a nonthreatening manner.

- Use a caring tone of voice and facial expression to help alleviate the client's fears.
- Speak slowly and distinctly, but not loudly.
- Conduct the interview in an unhurried manner.
- Follow acceptable social and cultural amenities.
- Ask general questions during the information-gathering stage.
- Be patient when the respondent gives information that seems unrelated to the client's health problem.
- Develop a trusting relationship by listening carefully, allowing time, and giving the client your full attention.
- Use gestures and pictures to help the client understand.
- Repeat the message in different ways if necessary.

Step 7 Use interpreters to improve communication.

- Ask the interpreter to translate the message, not just the individual words.
- Obtain feedback to confirm understanding.
- Use an interpreter who is culturally sensitive.

Communicating With the Angry Client

Responding to an angry client can be especially challenging. However, there are strategies, like these that follow, that can be used to defuse most situations*:

- Be aware of nonverbal communication. Do not rush, demand, react with hostility, or be overly cheerful. Be calm, move slowly, avoid touch, and maintain eye contact and a firm body posture. A client who is losing control is frightened. A nurse's appearance of control without rigidity is reassuring.
- Validate the presence of anger if possible. Say, "I understand why you may be angry." If you use a reflective statement such as "You seem angry," you may receive an angry response. Don't accentuate the obvious, but validate gently.
- Do not shut the door on anger. Explaining too soon, justifying yourself, or reassuring before the client can vent anger is not helpful and only serves to escalate anger. Do not condescend ("Tell me about it; I want to help") or interpret ("You are angry because I'm an authority figure"). Do not pass the buck or pretend to be unaccountable ("Wait for the physician" or "It's not my fault"). Anger is a feeling, not logical reasoning.
- Listen for the cause and meaning of the client's anger. There may be a reasonable explanation for the anger, and the solution may be self-evident. Help the client locate the source and meaning of the anger. Has the client lost his or her perceived control? self-esteem? autonomy? role? Most often, an angry client has lost, or believes he or she will lose, something of value.
- Search for a solution to the situation using problem-solving methods.
- If the client's anger continues to escalate, the nurse may want to offer a "time-out" or medication, explaining to the client that anger is permissible but loss of control is not. A quiet environment or medication may promote calmness. A nurse must protect the client and him- or herself from harm and minimize destruction of property. Limit-setting often pro-

*Adapted from Beare PG and Myers JL: *Principles and practice of adult health nursing, ed. 2*, St. Louis, 1994, Mosby-Year Book, Inc.

vides structure to the client's experience and lowers the energy that accompanies anger.

■ Refrain from showing fear. When nurses perceive their own anxiety, they require help.

■ Talk about the episode of anger after the client regains calmness. Teach the client the interplay between anxiety and anger, look for different ways the situation could be handled, role play, and support the client. Angry clients must not be rejected.

Communicating Effectively With Older Clients

Communicating with older clients often requires extra time and patience because of physical, psychologic, and social changes of normal aging. The following tips make communication with older people easier*:

■ Before you begin your conversation, reduce distratcting background noises (turn off the radio or television, close the door, move to a quieter place).

■ Begin the conversation with casual topics (the weather, what the person had for lunch). Avoid crucial messages at the beginning.

■ Continue conversation with familiar subjects such as family members and special interests of the person.

■ Stick to a topic for a while. Avoid quick shifts from topic to topic.

■ Keep your sentences and questions short. Rephrase rather than repeat a misunderstood sentence.

■ Give older persons a chance to reminisce. Their memories are important to them.

■ Allow extra time for responding. As people age, they function better at a slower tempo. Do not hurry them.

■ Give the person choices to ease decision making ("Do you want tea or coffee?" rather than "What do you want to drink?").

■ Be an active listener. If you are not sure what is being said, look for hints from eye gaze and gestures. Then take a guess ("Are you talking about the television news? Yes? Tell me more. I didn't see it.").

*From the American Speech, Language and Hearing Association, Rockville, Md, 1988.

Client Education

Self-care instruction for home care shares many of the challenges associated with client education in any situation. In home care, however, an important difference is control of the environment. Since the nurse is a guest in the client's home, he or she has less control than in other settings.

The home health nurse serves as both facilitator and collaborator for clients and caregivers as they assume primary responsibility for care and make decisions about the best methods for accomplishing treatment goals. This can be accomplished only in a spirit of mutual respect and sharing (LaRocca, 1994).

Special circumstances that must be taken into account in the education of clients and families in the home include the following*:

- Home health care requires the client's active participation in treatment. The client or caregiver must achieve a sense of control and mastery over the care. Consistent, understandable information is an important factor in making this happen.
- The stress of hospitalization or the physician's office setting as well as the client's anxiety over current physical conditions may limit his or her ability to remember important information presented in these settings. The client's or caregiver's understanding of treatment information and self-care skills must be reevaluated in the home environment.
- Often clients have been exposed to a large team of professionals, some with conflicting concerns and perspectives. Home health nurses must determine what already has been taught and continue to coordinate the approach for home health care.

A structured teaching program is required to meet initial home care learning needs. The amount of follow-up instruction must be individualized according to complexity of information and caregiver skill level. The client or caregiver must be taught to play an active role in assessing and reporting all problems. Before a client or caregiver can be independent in providing self-care, an understanding of the following information and skills is essential (LaRocca, 1994):

- Infection control
- Use of equipment
- Restricted activities

*LaRocca JC: *Handbook of home care IV therapy*, St. Louis, 1994, Mosby-Year Book, Inc.

- Medication schedule and administration
- Recognition and prevention of side effects
- Identification of emergency situations

Types of Learners

People learn in a variety of ways, usually favoring one method over another. There are, essentially, four kinds of learners: visual, auditory, tactile, and combination. Some individuals' learning strategies vary from situation to situation, depending on a number of external factors, although studies would suggest that they usually tend to have one method of learning that remains most effective for them under normal circumstances. Table 6 lists the four basic kinds of learners and the strategies most effective for each.

Table 6   Learning Strategies for Different Kinds of Learners

Types of Learners	Most Effective Strategy
Visual	Benefits most from written instructions and visual demonstrations. Video instruction is often helpful.
Auditory	Benefits most from verbal explanations and instruction. Video instruction is often helpful.
Tactile	Benefits most from hands-on instruction; learns best how to perform a procedure by actually doing it.
Combination	Benefits most from either visual, auditory, or tactile methods or tools, depending on the learning situation.

Adult Learning Principles

The following principles should be kept in mind when planning educational activities for adult clients*:

- Learning is an active process and adults prefer to participate actively. When you interact with your clients during an information-giving session, they will remember a lot more of what you said.
- Learning is goal-directed and adults are trying to satisfy a need. The information people want and need is in direct relation to their lives as they see it and the way they want to resume living. The most often asked question is, "How much can I do?" No matter why people are confined to their homes, they almost always feel that recovery is directly related to how much they do or don't do.
- Learning that is applied immediately is retained longer and is more subject to immediate use than that which is not. For example, when teaching clients about insulin, if you allow them to check their own glucose level and administer their own insulin under your supervision, you enable them to feel comfortable doing it themselves in their homes.
- Learning must be reinforced. Reinforcement means repetition. Clients have a need to hear the same explanation and advice from different sources. This applies especially to a person who has difficulty grasping or believing a concept.
- Learning new material is facilitated when it is related to what is already known. Build on what your clients already know. Find out what your clients' perceptions of recovery are and fill in what is missing in order to help them understand their role in their own care.
- The existence of periodic plateaus in the rate of learning necessitates frequent changes in teaching methods to ensure continuous progress. People can absorb only so much at one time. They also learn in different ways, so using different teaching methods will enhance learning.
- Learning is facilitated when the learner is aware of his or her progress. If clients realize that they have made progress in what they need to know to take care of themselves, they feel good about themselves and are willing to learn more.

*Adapted from Winthrop E: *Client teaching tips*, in *Mosby's Patient Teaching Guides*, St. Louis, 1995, Mosby-Year Book, Inc.

■ Learning is facilitated when there is a logic to the subject matter and the logic makes sense in relation to the learner's repertoire of experience. The way you can apply this principle is to ask people what their experience is with a particular illness.

Guidelines for Effective Education

Many factors affect learning in any situation. Some considerations include the following*:

■ Be sure you are skilled in presenting information in an understandable, orderly manner.

■ Be sure that information is presented in a way that meets the client's learning style.

■ Be sure that the client or caregiver is ready and able to learn.

■ If possible, ask the client to help you determine any learning needs. While respecting the favored learning methods of the client, keep in mind that most of us are "combination" learners. Do not rely only on verbal or printed instructions.

■ Point out important information in pamphlets and highlight this material for the client; say something like, "This is a key point." Written instructions are most effective when combined with discussion and demonstration.

■ Select a location for instruction that is as free from distraction as possible yet allows for inclusion of all support persons in the instruction; speak slowly when giving instructions.

■ Divide information into essential and nonessential elements, and initially teach only what is essential.

■ Emphasize what to do rather than what not to do. Avoid long explanations.

■ Have the client restate instructions as the procedure is being demonstrated, providing immediate feedback and praise.

■ Demonstrate each procedure and then watch the client perform the procedure. Coach the client to perform procedures correctly.

■ Do not suggest alternative procedures until a routine is established.

A popular strategy is to implement flow sheets for the client to use as a tool for effective self-care and to assist the nurse in monitoring compliance. It is also helpful to elicit suggestions from the client or caregiver when they experience difficulty following

*Adapted from LaRocca JC: *Handbook of home care IV therapy*, St. Louis, 1994, Mosby-Year Book, Inc.

the prescribed regimen. Listening to the client's suggestions and preferences will help make the treatment program successful. Try presenting personalized scenarios of complications and discussing actions that would be taken for each complication. Finally, always provide feedback, and encourage the client to practice while the nurse is present to supervise a new skill.

In addition, consider psychomotor, cognitive, and affective dimensions. All of us learn most easily when we believe that the information we've been asked to learn is perceived as logical, goals are achievable, and therapy is worthwhile. Not only does the client need to know enough to understand the care, but the client or caregiver must want to perform the care. For this reason, readiness to learn is best enhanced by addressing issues most important to the client first. Some important dimensions to consider include the following*:

- What has already been learned
- Client's and family's perception of the seriousness of the situation
- Emotional response to the illness
- Degree of support from family members
- Client's and caregiver's education and reading levels
- Amount of fatigue and discomfort
- Effects of medications and treatments
- Client's and caregiver's physical condition, including functional status, vision, hearing, fine motor skills, and cognitive abilities
- Any deficits in short-term memory
- Family's social support system and methods of dealing with stress, including cultural factors such as male/female role relationships, age, and country of origin

Sources of Tension in Client Education

The client's age, literacy skills, and family dynamics are three of the most common factors—outside the client's physical condition—that can interfere with the effectiveness of home health care. Home care creates stress and often forges new roles in the home. Family conflict can occur when client care requires a disproportionate amount of family time or resources and when information is not shared with all family members. Table 7 offers some helpful responses to some of the most common sources of tension in client and family/caregiver education (LaRocca, 1994).

*LaRocca JC: *Handbook of home care IV therapy*, St. Louis, 1994, Mosby-Year Book, Inc.

Table 7 Relieving External Tensions in Client and Family Education

Problem	Response
Family Dynamics	
Client or family member feels overwhelmed	Goalsetting: Help family refocus on tasks at hand. Review goals that have been attained to boost morale.
Anxiety and fear of performing complex procedures	Establish an atmosphere of acceptance. Don't be in a hurry. Offer opportunities for talk and questions. Reassure client/family that they have made the right treatment choice.
Emotions associated with chronic or terminal conditions	Provide opportunities to express feelings. Offer referrals to community resources.
Caregiver burnout and illness	Simplify client management where possible (e.g., scheduling drug doses to reduce nighttime treatment). Remain accessible. Remember: When caregiver needs are not being met, resentments increase.
Client fatigue, especially with chronic illnesses	Help the client identify individual tolerance for tiredness in planning for as much active participation in the family life as possible.

(Continued)

Table 7   Relieving External Tensions in Client and Family Education (cont'd)

Problem	Response
Low Literacy Skills	
Increased difficulty in categorizing information; fewer generalizations between situations	Teach in concrete terms, using words already understood. Use simple line drawings and frequent repetition. Additional telephone checks help.
Geriatric Considerations	
An increase in the number of drugs taken daily (on average 4 or more a day) increases the potential for adverse reactions	Use only one pharmacy so that one source keeps track. Continually evaluate all drugs taken for need, safety, compatibility, potential adverse reactions, and expiration dates.
Frequently, decreased visual acuity	Use teaching materials with large, bold type. Encourage the use of a magnifying glass.
Pediatric Considerations	
Children are vulnerable to accidental poisoning	Remind families to store medications and supplies out of reach.
Decreased compliance with treatment and education	Emphasize the importance of taking medications on schedule. Use stickers to reward the compliant child. Stories and puppets are often effective with younger children.

(Continued)

Table 7 Relieving External Tensions in Client and Family Education (cont'd)

Problem	Response
Young clients are frequently overwhelmed by complex emotions about their illness and therapy.	Encourage both children and adolescents to use artwork to express their feelings.
	Offer support to parents and siblings who must alter the family lifestyle.

Adapted from LaRocca JC: *Handbook of home care IV therapy*, St. Louis, 1994, Mosby-Year Book, Inc.

Developing and Selecting Client Education Materials

The following materials and strategies enhance the education process*:
- Combinations of text and line drawings
- Procedures presented in order of performance
- Material organized according to importance, with the most important concepts presented first and/or last since first- and last-taught information is remembered longer
- Reading levels of approximately sixth to ninth grade for most clients
- Short words and short sentences
- A conversational writing style in the active voice (e.g., "Clean the port with an alcohol wipe.")
- Consistent terms (e.g., "IV catheter" and "IV line")
- Focusing on what readers should do, not what they should not do: "Use only medications that are clear," rather than "Do not use medications that are cloudy"
- Good print quality, with strong color contrasts to assist people with limited vision, and paper that does not produce a glare

LaRocca JC: *Handbook of home care IV therapy*, St. Louis, 1994, Mosby-Year Book, Inc.

- Audiotapes that review printed material
- Good lighting

Special Documentation Considerations for Client Teaching

Document all aspects of client and caregiver education, including the following (LaRocca, 1994):

- Topic of education
- Assessment of retained learning
- All activities involved in teaching, including teaching aids used
- Ability of the client and caregiver to learn and understand
- All reteaching that is required and the reason

Client Rights

The Patient's Bill of Rights and the Patient Self-Determination Act delineate the essential rights of all clients regardless of the setting in which they receive health care.

Patient's Bill of Rights

Home health agencies, like all other health facilities, must protect and promote the rights of each individual under their care. Like nurses in other health fields, home health nurses are responsible for protecting the client according to the Patient's Bill of Rights from the American Hospital Association (AHA). These rights are as follows*:

- The patient has the right to considerate and respectful care.
- The patient has the right to and is encouraged to obtain from physicians and other direct caregivers relevant, current, and understandable information concerning diagnosis, treatment, and prognosis.

  Except in emergencies when the patient lacks decision-making capacity and the need for treatment is urgent, the patient is entitled to the opportunity to discuss and request information related to the specific procedures and/or treatments, the risks involved, the possible length of recuperation, and the medically reasonable alternatives and their accompanying risks and benefits.
- Patients have the right to know the identity of physicians, nurses, and others involved in their care, as well as when those involved are students, residents, or other trainees. The patient also has the right to know the immediate and long-term financial implications of treatment choices, insofar as they are known.
- The patient has the right to make decisions about the plan of care prior to and during the course of treatment and to refuse a recommended treatment or plan of care to the extent permitted by law and hospital policy and to be informed of the medical consequences of this action. In case of such refusal, the patient is entitled to other appropriate care and services that the hospital provides or transfer to another hospital. The hospital should notify patients of any policy

*© 1992 by the American Hospital Association, Chicago, Illinois. Used with permission.

that might affect patient choice within the institution.

- The patient has the right to have an advance directive (such as a living will, health care proxy, or durable power of attorney for health care) concerning treatment or designating a surrogate decision maker with the expectation that the hospital will honor the intent of that directive to the extent permitted by law and hospital policy. Health care institutions must advise patients of their rights under state law and hospital policy to make informed medical choices, ask if the patient has an advance directive, and include that information in patient records. The patient has the right to timely information about hospital policy that may limit its ability to implement fully a legally valid advance directive.
- The patient has the right to every consideration of privacy. Case discussion, consultation, examination, and treatment should be conducted so as to protect each patient's privacy.
- The patient has the right to expect that all communications and records pertaining to his or her care will be treated as confidential by the hospital, except in cases such as suspected abuse and public health hazards when reporting is permitted or required by law. The patient has the right to expect that the hospital will emphasize the confidentiality of this information when it releases it to any other parties entitled to review information in these records.
- The patient has the right to review the records pertaining to his or her medical care and to have the information explained or interpreted as necessary, except when restricted by law.
- The patient has the right to expect that, within its capacity and policies, a hospital will make reasonable response to the request of a patient for appropriate and medically indicated care and services. The hospital must provide evaluation, service, and/or referral as indicated by the urgency of the case. When medically appropriate and legally permissible, or when a patient has so requested, a patient may be transferred to another facility. The institution to which the patient is to be transferred must first have accepted the patient for transfer. The patient must also have the benefit of complete information and explanation concerning the need for, risks and benefits of, and alternatives to such a transfer.
- The patient has the right to ask and be informed of the existence of business relationships among the hospital, educational institutions, other health care providers, or payers that may influence the patient's treatment and care.

- The patient has the right to consent to or decline to participate in proposed research studies or human experimentation affecting care and treatment or requiring direct patient involvement, and to have those studies fully explained prior to consent. A patient who declines to participate in research or experimentation is entitled to the most effective care that the hospital can otherwise provide.
- The patient has the right to expect reasonable continuity of care when appropriate and to be informed by physicians and other caregivers of available and realistic patient care options when hospital care is no longer appropriate.
- The patient has the right to be informed of hospital policies and practices that relate to patient care, treatment, and responsibilities. The patient has the right to be informed of available resources for resolving disputes, grievences, and conflicts, such as ethics committees, patient representatives, or other mechanisms available in the institution. The patient has the right to be informed of the hospital's charges for services and available payment methods.

Guidelines for Patient Self-Determination

The Patient Self-Determination Act (PSDA) was incorporated into the Omnibus Budget Reconciliation Act of 1990 (OBRA 1990) and took effect December 1, 1991. This act essentially mandates that health care facilities are responsible for ensuring that individuals enrolled in their facilities are informed of their right to formulate advance directives and their right to consent to or refuse treatment.

An advance directive is a written statement of how one wants medical decisions made. It allows the individual to make choices for health care or to designate someone to make those choices if the individual is unable to make decisions about medical treatment now or in the future. It allows that individual to say "yes" to treatment wanted or "no" to treatment not wanted (Jaffe & Skidmore-Roth, 1993).

Types of Advance Directives

Living will. A living will is a written form, approved by the writer's state, that specifies the kind of medical care the writer wants or does not want if he or she becomes unable to make his or her own decisions. A living will may be initiated by using a form developed by the state, completing and signing a preprinted form available in the community, developing one's own form, or writing a statement of treatment preferences. Advice may be solicited from an attorney or physician to ensure that one's wishes are understood and followed.

Durable power of attorney for health care. This document is a signed, dated, and witnessed paper naming another person, such as a spouse, child, or close friend, as the client's agent or proxy to make medical decisions for the client if he or she should become unable to make them for himself or herself. The document may include instructions about any treatment the client wishes to avoid. Some states have specific laws allowing for health care power of attorney and provide preprinted forms.

Depending on state laws, it may be preferable to have either a living will or a durable power of attorney for health care, and it may be possible to have both or to combine the two types in a document that describes treatment choices in situations and names someone to make decisions for the client when necessary. Either of these may be changed or canceled at any time. Some states allow a change by oral statement.

An advance directive should be signed and dated, with copies given to the physician and others as needed. A copy should be given to the client's attorney if he or she has a durable power of attorney; a copy should also be given to the physician to become a part of the permanent record. Finally, a copy should be put in a safe place where it can be found easily if needed. A card should be placed in the client's purse or wallet that states the existence of an advance directive, where it is located, and the name of the client's agent or proxy if appropriate (Jaffe & Skidmore-Roth, 1993).

This legislation affects virtually all health care facilities participating in Medicare and Medicaid programs: hospitals, nursing homes, home health agencies, hospices, and health maintenance organizations. These agencies are required to:

- Provide education to the staff regarding these issues.
- Maintain written policies and procedures for adherence to these requirements.
- Ensure that the medical record reflects the client's status regarding advance directives.
- Not discriminate against any client on the basis of individual decision making regarding advance directives.

To ensure that the legislation addresses the problem as it was intended, home health nurses need to see that clients and their surrogates are aware of their right to formulate choices for the withholding or withdrawal of treatment under prespecified conditions.

Home Health Nursing Guidelines for Advance Directives

Home health nurses need to*:

- Formulate advance directives themselves.
- Assist in determining a client's competency when there is reason to doubt it.
- Ensure that the client and family have sufficient information about the state statutes and the PSDA itself to make any desired decisions.
- Recognize that not all individuals are ready to make decisions.
- Be prepared to act on the client's behalf if necessary.
- Recognize the emotional state of the client's family and help them to come to terms with the client's advance directive formulated as a result of PSDA.
- Ensure that agency administration has provided detailed policies and procedures, as well as thorough and comprehensive education of the individuals responsible for enforcing this statute.
- Facilitate discussions so that the involved individuals recognize that they are involved in a decision-making process, not a death-producing process.
- Ensure that formative, summative, and ongoing evaluation mechanisms are in place in terms of implementation methodologies for enforcing the PSDA.
- Serve and be active on ethics committees, or if necessary, establish one.
- Ensure that no client is discriminated against regarding type or quality of health care for any reason.
- Ensure that whatever the client's decision, it was not coerced; decisions must be strictly voluntary and reflect the individual's values, desires, and wishes.

To help in determining the competency of a client, the following five questions should be considered (Weber, 1993):

- Can the client receive (hear or read) information?
- Can the client process and comprehend information?
- Can the client appropriately assess the relevant information?
- Can the client use relevant information to make a decision?
- Can the client make a decision and give a reason for it?

*Adapted from Weber G: *Tips on implementing the patient self-determination act*, excerpted with permission from Nursing and Health Care, Vol. 14, Number 2, © 1993, National League for Nursing.

Assessment

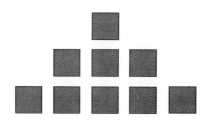

Assessment and History*

Admission and Client History

The client history and symptom assessment serves as a guide for the physical examination, establishes a baseline from which to assess changes over time, and helps to determine priorities for the plan of care. A detailed history may or may not be provided with the home care referral; therefore it may be necessary for the nurse to obtain one during the initial visits.

The client is the primary source of information for the history, although valuable information can be obtained from family members and caregivers as well.

Effective questioning and careful listening are important so that the client is at ease as the necessary information is gathered. Specific questions are organized by problem or physiologic system. Two or three home visits may be required before all of the historical data can be gathered. Whenever possible, a history, treatment plan, and hospital discharge summary should be obtained from the referring physician.

The admission client history needs to be taken only once and is useful when making referrals. The background information gathered will be helpful when performing the physical assessment. This and the following pages in this section offer the home health nurse outlines of the most frequently used assessments for a variety of conditions. The first is a general, comprehensive health history (Jaffe & Skidmore-Roth, 1993).

Health History/Medications

Identifying Information
- Age, sex, race, ethnicity, marital status, children and ages
- Religious practices, cultural influences
- Occupation
- Educational level
- Health insurance
- Residence
- Source of information

*All assessments provided in this section are from Jaffe MS and Skidmore-Roth L: *Home health nursing care plans, ed. 2*, St. Louis, 1993, Mosby-Year Book, Inc.

- Referred by
- Reliability of informant
- Doctor's name, address

Chief Complaint

- Ask, "What specific problem caused you to seek help today?" (Record as a quote exactly what the client says)
- Ask, "How long has this been a problem?"

Detailed History of Illness

- What: What were you doing at the time the problem occurred?
- When: When did it begin (date, time of day)?
- How: Was it a recurring or sudden onset? Severity?
- Why: Did any precipitating events occur?

Past Health History

- Statement about general health
- Other major medical conditions (diabetes, cardiac) and dates of onset or occurrence
- Hospitalizations
- Surgeries and injuries and dates
- Military history, travel, and dates
- Childhood diseases and ages at which they occurred
- Psychiatric illness and treatment
- Usual health care patterns and kind of practitioner used
- Use of rehabilitative/support personnel
- Lifestyle patterns and personal habits in sleep, nutrition, fluid intake, urinary and bowel elimination, activity, sexual behavior, personal hygiene, and others
- Allergies
- Immunizations
- Habits: caffeine, alcohol, drugs, and cigarettes
- Present medications (including over-the-counter)
- Nutrition, diet, weight loss or gain
- Significant family illness or death

Medications/Treatments

- Oxygen use
- Street or recreational drug use
- Homeotherapy
- Over-the counter drugs: type, frequency, dosage, length of use, side effects, desired effect and condition(s) being treated, how taken, drug form, contraindications

- Potential for toxicity
- Aids used to ensure safe, correct administration
- Effect of client's age on absorption and excretion
- Treatment for adverse effects

Present History

- Chief complaint (in client's words, if possible)
- Onset and development of problems, where took place, what was done
- Signs and symptoms and their location, severity, duration, and frequency; changes and effect on client; meaning of disease to client
- Factors that alleviated or aggravated symptoms
- Client's knowledge of disease, procedures, and planned therapy
- Client's adaptation to disorder if chronic
- Laboratory and diagnostic tests done during hospitalization
- Medications and treatments since discharge
- Homebound status

Psychosocial History

- Consumption of coffee, alcohol or tobacco; amount, frequency, and type
- General appearance
- Living arrangements, significant persons and relations with them
- Occupation and income, ability to pay for health care (Medicare, Medicaid, CHAMPUS, private insurance, Workers' Compensation)
- Education, degrees, profession if applicable
- Recreation and interests; retirement if applicable
- Friends, community involvement, church activities
- English as a second language or no English spoken
- Emergency contact and telephone number

Family History

- Health status of parents, spouse, siblings, and children, including deaths with ages and causes
- Health status of grandparents and other blood relatives
- Roles and responsibilities of family members and whether they work outside the home
- Relationships with family members, activities, response to stress or crisis
- History of abuse by family members or relatives

- Marital relationship
- Family members' history of heart conditions, diabetes, cancer, or other diseases
- Adaptation of family members to care of client in the home

Review of Systems

Vital Signs

- Height, weight, temperature, blood pressure

Pulmonary System

- Chronic obstructive pulmonary disease (COPD); pneumonia; upper respiratory infection; influenza; throat infections; pain in throat, nose, or chest; congestion of or discharge from nose; epistaxis; hemoptysis; cough and sputum with characteristics; dyspnea with or without exertion; wheezing; abnormal breath sounds

Cardiovascular System

- Chest pain; arm, throat, or jaw pain; edema; dyspnea; palpitations; hypertension; phlebitis; diminished circulation to extremities; heart condition; claudication; paresthesia

Neurologic System

- Headaches, fainting, seizures, tremors, dizziness, paralysis, changes in sensory perception (touch, taste, smell, vision, hearing), mentation changes, use of glasses or contact lenses, hearing aid, motor changes (gait, coordination), sleep/rest patterns, speech

Gastrointestinal System

- Hepatitis; diverticulosis; gallstones; peptic ulcer; colitis; ostomy; cirrhosis; abdominal pain; nausea; vomiting; diarrhea; constipation; hemorrhoids; indigestion; swallowing; anorexia; excessive flatus, belching, or eructation; changes in stool color, consistency, or frequency; chewing problems; presence of dentures and fit; 24-hour dietary intake; special diets

Endocrine System

- Diabetes, thyroid condition, polyuria, polydipsia, appetite, tolerance of heat or cold, Cushing's syndrome

Hematologic System

- Anemia; skin hemorrhages, bruising, or petechiae; previous transfusions; bleeding from any site; weakness; pallor; night sweats

Musculoskeletal System

- Fractures; arthritis; osteoporosis; pain or stiffness in joints; redness, swelling, or heat in joints; limited range of motion (ROM); fatigue; weakness or pain in muscles; assistive devices; ability to perform activities of daily living (ADL)

Renal/Urinary Systems

- Difficulty in urination, dysuria, dribbling, incontinence, urgency, frequency, retention, hematuria, calculi, urinary tract infections (UTI), glomerulonephritis, prostatic hypertrophy, chronic renal failure, fluid intake/output for 24 hours

Integumentary System

- Rash; pruritis; lesions; change in skin color, nails, or hair; scar tissue; dryness; oiliness

Reproductive System

- Lesions on or drainage from penis or vulva; rashes or irritations on penis or vulva; vaginal infections; sexually transmitted disease; infertility; use of birth control; sexual pattern and satisfaction or difficulties; age at menarche and menopause; abnormal vaginal bleeding or menstrual irregularity; number of pregnancies, live births, and abortions; complications of pregnancy; impotence; last menstrual period (LMP); last Pap smear, mammogram, and breast examination; lumps or pain in breasts; discharge from breasts; penile implant

Psychiatric

- Depression, nervousness, chronic anxiety, or worry; mood swings; decreased self-concept; effect of stress; thoughts of suicide; hallucinations, delusions, or paranoid manifestations

Physical Assessment*

Pulmonary System Assessment

Past History

Lung and Airway Disorders

- Bronchitis
- Asthma
- Emphysema
- Tuberculosis
- Pneumonia
- Pleurisy, pleural effusion
- Lung malignancy
- Influenza and colds and frequency
- Chest surgery or injury

Signs and Symptoms of Respiratory Distress

- Dyspnea with or without exertion, breathlessness
- Coughing and sneezing: amount and frequency
- Sputum: amount, consistency, and color
- Chest pain
- Wheezing

Family History

- Respiratory disorders: acute or chronic
- Allergies, eczema

Allergies

- Plants
- Animals
- Foods
- Drugs
- Environmental pollutants

Immunizations

- Pneumonia
- Influenza

Activities of Daily Living (ADL)

- Position during sleep for optimal breathing

*All assessments provided in this section are from Jaffe MS and Skidmore-Roth L: *Home health nursing care plans, ed. 2*, St. Louis, 1993, Mosby-Year Book, Inc.

- Amount of exercise and effects on breathing
- Abilities for personal self-care and/or ADL
- Homebound status

Psychosocial History

- Tobacco consumption: amount and duration of use
- Alcohol consumption
- Personality traits, anxiety
- Home environment and exposure to irritants (odors, smoke, sprays, allergens, air conditioning, humidity)
- Adaptation to illness or chronic condition

Past Treatments and Diagnostic Procedures

- Desensitization therapy
- Medications (prescribed and OTC) taken for respiratory or other conditions
- Breathing treatments (nebulizer, physiotherapy, breathing exercises)
- Lung biopsy, thoracentesis, bronchoscopy
- Chest x-ray studies, pulmonary function studies, sputum culture, laboratory tests for drug levels and arterial blood gas levels (ABGs)
- Past or recent hospitalizations

Present History

Chief Complaint, Including Onset and Length of Time Present

Signs and Symptoms

- Respiratory rate, ease, and depth; factors precipitating increases or other changes
- Dyspnea, orthopnea, tachypnea
- Chest pain
- Fatigue, activity intolerance
- Cyanosis, pallor
- Productive or nonproductive cough and characteristics (amount, color, consistency)
- Use of accessory muscles

Knowledge of Disease and Planned Home Therapy

Present Treatments and Diagnostic Procedures

- Laboratory and diagnostic tests and results
- Use of oxygen
- Medications (oral, inhalants)

- Bronchodilators
- Sedatives
- Steroids
- Tranquilizers
- Others

Physical Examination

Inspection

- Symmetry of chest (shape, expansion, movement)
- Color of lips, ears, and nails
- Breathing pattern using mouth, diaphragm, chest, and abdomen; use of accessory muscles
- Nail bed capillary refill
- Clubbing of fingers
- Confusion
- Fatigue
- Restlessness
- Diaphoresis

Palpation

- Chest for pain or masses
- Skin for warmth, dryness, and smoothness
- Intercostal muscles for firmness, smoothness, bulging, and retraction
- Vocal and tactile fremitus and location of increases or decreases
- Symmetry of anterior and posterior chest expansion

Percussion

- Lung field resonance: hyperresonance, dull sound, flatness, and tympany
- Pitch, intensity, duration (anteriorly and posteriorly with bilateral comparison)

Auscultation

- Voice sounds for intensity at airways and periphery
- Adventitious sounds such as rales, rhonchi, wheezes, and stridor; note position in lungs (1/2, 1/4, bases)
- Normal breath sounds such as bronchial, tracheal, vesicular, bronchovesicular, whether diminished or absent, and location
- Breath sounds heard in areas where not expected (abnormal)

Cardiovascular System Assessment

Past History

Cardiovascular Disorders

- Hypertension
- Congestive heart failure
- Stroke
- Coronary artery disease
- Myocardial infarction
- Thrombophlebitis
- Leg ulcer, varicose veins
- Arterial insufficiency
- Heart surgery (bypass, valvular)

Signs and Symptoms of Cardiac or Vascular Distress

- Pain in chest, arms, throat, jaw, or extremities
- Heart palpitations
- Dyspnea, orthopnea, cough
- Neck vein distention
- Edema
- Cold, numbness, or tingling of extremities
- Discoloration of extremities
- Dizziness, weakness

Family History

- Heart or vascular condition: acute or chronic
- Hypertension
- Coronary heart disease
- Diabetes mellitus
- Asthma
- Stroke
- Obesity

Allergies

- Medications
- Foods

Activities of Daily Living (ADL)

- Sleeping with head elevated
- Abilities for personal self-care and/or ADL
- Exercising and effect on pulse and respiration
- Homebound status
- Special diet: low-cholesterol/fat, low-sodium, or low-calorie

Psychosocial History

- Tobacco, caffeine, and alcohol consumption: daily and over period of years
- Personality traits
- Occupation and work-related stress
- Adaptation to illness or chronic condition

Past Treatments and Diagnostic Procedures

- Pacemaker insertion
- Holter monitor
- Medications (prescribed and OTC) taken for heart or other conditions
- Cardiac rehabilitation
- Electrocardiogram, echocardiogram, angiogram, cardiac catheterization, x-ray studies, stress test
- Laboratory tests for enzymes, lipid panel, electrolytes, and prothrombin time
- Cardiac or vascular surgery
- Angioplasty, laser treatments
- Past or recent hospitalizations

Present History

Chief Complaint, Including Onset and Length of Time Present

Signs and Symptoms

- Blood pressure; pulse rate (beats/min) and regularity: apical pulse; factors that cause changes in baselines: changes with position or posture (sitting, standing, lying)
- Onset, duration, precipitating factors if any, alleviating factors if relevant
- Chest, arm, throat, or jaw pain; aching in legs; pain in leg calf; edema and/or redness
- Dyspnea, orthopnea
- Palpitations
- Edema, weight gain
- Changes in pulse rate (slow or rapid) and regularity
- Change in mentation: headache
- Insomnia, restlessness, fatigue
- Changes in skin color (pallor, redness, cyanosis)

Knowledge of Disease and Planned Home Therapy

Present Treatments and Diagnostic Procedures

- Laboratory and diagnostic tests and results
- Use of oxygen
- Medications (oral, sublingual)
  - Antihypertensives
  - Vasodilators
  - Cardiotonics
  - Diuretics
  - Anticoagulants
  - Aspirin
  - Nitrates
  - Others

Physical Examination

Inspection

- Symmetry of chest, legs, and arms
- Pulsations in the aortic area, pulmonary area, right-ventricular area, and apical or left-ventricular area
- Skin of arms, hands, legs, and feet for color and texture (pink, warm, smooth, dry); color change in extremities when dangling or elevated (should return to normal in 10 seconds)
- Hair distribution on legs and arms; clubbing of fingers
- Rashes, scars, ulcers, exudate and discoloration (brownish color, eschar, irregular shape of ulcer, chronic venous stasis)
- Veins flush with skin surface or venous enlargement
- Capillary refill of nail beds of less than 3 seconds

Palpation

- Skin of extremities smooth, dry, and warm to touch
- Masses in extremities or chest
- Pain or tenderness in chest or extremities
- Veins smooth and full or dilated and tortuous
- Cardiac thrills (pulsations of the heart that feel like the throat of a purring cat)
- Radial pulse rate and characteristics
- Femoral popliteal, carotid temporal, and dorsalis pedis pulse rates and characteristics
- Apical pulse, point of maximum impulse (PMI), and other areas of pulsations of the heart
- Edema in legs: dependent or pitting
- Calf for signs of phlebitis (tenderness, tension)
- Homans' sign: present or absent

Auscultation

- Apical and radial pulses, noting rate, regularity, and pulse deficit
- Apical pulse, noting rate, regularity, and intensity
- Blood pressure, using brachial artery and noting Korotkoff signs and pulse pressure
- Heart sounds (S_1 and S_2), extra heart sounds (S_3 and S_4)
- Murmur, noting timing, location, and sound distribution
- Clicks and snaps, noting timing, intensity, and pitch
- Friction rub
- Carotid artery for bruits

Neurologic System Assessment

Past History

Neurologic Motor and Sensory Disorders

- Multiple sclerosis
- Muscular dystrophy
- Cerebrovascular accident (CVA)
- Seizure disorder
- Head trauma
- Spinal cord injury
- Motor or sensory aberrations
- Parkinson's disease
- Hearing, vision, and speech impairments
- Surgeries (craniotomy, laminectomy)

Signs and Symptoms of Neurologic Disease

- Headaches
- Tremors
- Paralysis
- Gait disturbance
- Mental retardation
- Behavioral changes (confusion, disorientation, mood, affect)
- Speech changes
- Mentation changes
- Seizure activity

Family History

- Neurologic disorders: acute or chronic
- Hypertension
- Stroke

- Epilepsy
- Alzheimer s disease, dementia
- Huntington's chorea
- Diabetes mellitus

Allergies

- Medications

Activities of Daily Living (ADL)

- Abilities for personal self-care and/or ADL
- Amount of independence or dependence
- Rest/sleep/nap patterns (hours/24 hours; frequency; times; length; use and effect of sleeping aids, prescribed or OTC; factors that promote or prevent sleep)
- Homebound status

Psychosocial History

- Drug, alcohol, and tobacco consumption: daily and over period of years
- Occupational exposure to toxic agents that affect mental functioning
- Personality traits
- Adaptation to illness or chronic condition

Past Treatments and Diagnostic Procedures

- Medications (prescribed or OTC) taken for neurologic or other conditions
- Cerebral angiogram, lumbar puncture, scans, myogram ocular studies, blood flow studies, magnetic resonance imaging (MRI), electroencephalogram (EEG), skull or spinal x-ray studies
- Laboratory tests for electrolyte panel and cultures (cerebrospinal fluid, blood)
- Cranial or spinal surgery
- Past or recent hospitalizations

Present History

Chief Complaint, Including Onset, Length of Time Present, and Precipitating Factors

Signs and Symptoms

- Anxiety
- Sleep pattern changes, insomnia
- Headaches, back pain, dizziness

- Memory deficits: changes in level of consciousness and behavior
- Sensory problems (paresthesias)
- Motor problems (imbalance, paralysis, tic)
- Quadriplegia, paraplegia
- Fatigue, mood, and communication problems
- Aggressive behavior

Knowledge of Disease and Planned Home Therapy

Present Treatments and Diagnostic Procedures

- Laboratory and diagnostic tests and results
- Medications (oral)
  - Sedatives
  - Hypnotics
  - Narcotic and nonnarcotic analgesics
  - Tranquilizers
  - Antidepressants
  - Anticonvulsants
  - Others

Physical Examination

Inspection

- Vital signs, including temperature
- Motor function (gait, coordination, balance, tremors during rest or intentional, ataxia, speech difficulty, dysphagia, symmetry of muscle size, loss of muscle mass, muscle tone for spasticity and flaccidity, muscle strength in upper and lower extremities, involuntary muscle movements, range of motion in all joints)
- Sensory function (touch, pain, proprioception, vision, hearing, discriminatory sensation, temperature)
- Mental function (level of consciousness; orientation to time, place, and person; memory attention span; ability to make judgments and problem solve; ability to communicate; anger; agitation; euphoria; depression; lability)
- General appearance (posture, personal hygiene, facial expression)

Spinal Nerve Innervation
  - C-4: Motor function from neck downward
  - C-5: Raising of arms
  - C-5 through C-6: Flexion of elbow
  - C-6: Dorsiflexion of wrist

- C-7: Extension of elbow
- C-8: Flexion of finger
- T-1: Abduction of finger
- T-l through T-8: Movement of thoracic musculature
- T-6 through T-12: Movement of abdominal musculature
- L-1 through L-3: Flexion of hip
- L-2 through L-4: Extension of knee
- L-4 through L-5: Dorsiflexion of ankle
- L-5 through S-1: Extension of great toe
- S-1 through S-2: Plantar flexion of ankle
- S-3 through S-5: Movement of perianal muscle

Cranial Nerve Innervation

- Olfactory (sensory—smell): Odor identification, such as coffee, spice, or alcohol
- Optic (sensory—vision): Snellen chart for visual acuity; gross confrontation test; periphery test of four visual-field quadrants
- Oculomotor (motor—pupil constriction; eyelid and extraocular movements): Use penlight for pupil constriction; size and shape; ptosis of eyelid; accommodation to finger moving toward nose
- Trochlear (motor—eye movement inward and downward): Convergence of eyes inward when finger moves toward nose
- Trigeminal (motor—temporal, masseter muscles and lateral jaw movement; sensory—maxillary, mandibular facial and ophthalmic sensitivity): Movement of jaw and mastication muscles and ability to open and close jaws; sensitivity to sharp and dull object applied to each area with eyes closed; sensitivity of cornea to application of cotton wisp
- Abducent (motor—eye abduction): Eye muscle movement for disconjugate gaze; eyes not moving together
- Facial (motor—facial expressions; sensory—taste): Face and scalp muscle movement; grimacing; closing eyes tightly; discriminating salty and sweet tastes
- Acoustic (sensory—hearing with cochlear division and balance with vestibular division); Weber's and Rinne's tests for auditory acuity; balance testing done by physician
- Glossopharyngeal (motor—pharynx; sensory—taste and pharyngeal sensation): Swallowing ability and gag reflex; rise of uvula when saying "ah"; taste sensation at posterior tongue; hoarseness

- Vagus (motor—pharynx, larynx, palate; sensory—pharynx, larynx): Ability to speak and phonation; swallowing and gag reflex with nerve IX
- Spinal accessory (motor—sternocleidomastoid and trapezius muscle movements): Shoulder shrugging and turning head against resistance
- Hypoglossal (motor—tongue): Tongue protrusion, deviation, and strength

Palpation

- Symmetry, shape, masses, depressions of head and muscles
- Carotid and temporal pulses, comparing strength and quality bilaterally
- Muscles for tone, shape, size, and atrophy
- Skeletal muscle reflexes
  - Biceps and brachioradial (C-5, C-6)
  - Triceps (C-6, C-7, C-8)
  - Patellar (L-2, L-3, L-4)
  - Achilles (S-1, S-2)
  - Upper abdominal (T-8, T-9, T-10)
  - Lower abdominal (T-10, T-11, T-12)
  - Perineal or anal (S-3, S-4, S-5)
  - Cremasteric (L-1, L-2)

Auscultation

- Blood pressure
- Bruits over eyes, temples, and mastoid processes

Gastrointestinal System Assessment

Past History

Gastrointestinal Disorders

- Peptic ulcer
- Inflammatory bowel disease
- Diverticulosis
- Hepatitis
- Cirrhosis
- Enteritis
- Gallbladder disease
- Hemorrhoids
- Hernia
- Esophageal varices
- Gastrointestinal hemorrhage or surgery

Signs and Symptoms of Gastrointestinal Distress

- Nausea, vomiting
- Weight changes
- Anorexia
- Indigestion/heartburn
- Dysphagia
- Constipation
- Diarrhea
- Blood in vomitus or stool
- Abdominal pain/distention

Family History

- Gastrointestinal disorders: acute or chronic
- Ulcers
- Hemorrhoids
- Colorectal malignancies
- Hepatitis
- Obesity

Allergies

- Foods
- Medications

Patterns of Bowel Elimination and Nutrition Intake

- Characteristics, frequency, color, and amount of stool
- Increased flatus
- Laxatives or enemas used: type and frequency
- Food likes and dislikes, appetite, amount, frequency, ability to chew, dentures and denture pain
- Caloric intake (24-hour intake)
- Cultural influences
- Weight loss or gain/ideal body weight

Activities of Daily Living (ADL)

- Abilities for self-care (feeding and toileting)
- Special diet: low or high calorie
- Homebound status

Psychosocial History

- Tobacco, caffeine, and alcohol use: daily and over period of years
- Personality traits
- Stress and anxiety and effect on elimination and nutrition
- Adaptation to illness or chronic condition

Past Treatments and Diagnostic Procedures

- Presence of bowel diversion: type, care, and response
- Medications (prescribed and OTC) taken for gastrointestinal or other conditions
- Proctoscopy, gastroscopy, colonoscopy, scans, magnetic resonance imaging (MRI), stomach and bowel x-ray studies, gallbladder x-ray studies, liver biopsy
- Stool for occult blood, ova, parasites, toxins, and culture
- Gastrointestinal or mouth surgery
- Past or recent hospitalizations

Present History

Chief Complaint, Including Onset, Length of Time Present, and Severity

Signs and Symptoms

- Pain and characteristics
- Anorexia, nausea, vomiting
- Heartburn, flatulence, eructation
- Constipation, diarrhea, absence of bowel movements
- Weight changes
- Jaundice, pruritis
- Blood in vomitus or stool; black, tarry or chalky stool; coffee-ground vomitus

Knowledge of Disease and Planned Home Therapy

Present Treatment

- Diagnostic procedures and results
- Results of complete blood counts, electrolytes, blood urea nitrogen, bilirubin, lipase, amylase, and other laboratory tests
- Nasogastric tube feedings, total parenteral nutrition
- Gastric decompression, suctioning
- Enemas, bowel irrigation
- Medications (oral, rectal)
  - Vitamins
  - Antacids
  - Antiemetics
  - Antidiarrheals
  - H_2 antagonists
  - Laxatives, stool softeners, suppositories
  - Others

Physical Examination

Inspection
- Body contour, abdomen, umbilicus (shape, protrusion, size)
- Height and weight, noting amount over or under normal for age, size, sex, and frame
- Skin: rash, smoothness, scars, edema, and color
- Drainage from nasogastric tube or ostomy
- Stool and vomitus for abnormal constituents or consistency
- Mouth for pain, caries, dentures, stomatitis, lesions, bleeding, and odor
- Anus for pain, itching, inflammation, bleeding, and hemorrhoids
- Jaundice of skin, sclera, and mucous membranes

Palpation
- Abdominal masses, pain, nodes, distention, tautness, warmth, or coldness
- Skin turgor

Percussion
- Abdominal distention for dull, tympanic, or wavelike sounds
- Bladder distention for dull sounds

Auscultation
- Absence of bowel sounds for 5 minutes in four quadrants
- Presence of bowel sounds in four quadrants, including frequency, pitch, loudness, rushing, swishing, and gurgling

Endocrine System Assessment

Past History

Endocrine Disorders
- Diabetes mellitus
- Diabetes insipidus
- Addison's disease
- Hyperthyroidism or hypothyroidism
- Pituitary tumor
- Surgery (thyroidectomy)

Signs and Symptoms of Endocrine Disorders
- Weight changes, appetite and hydration changes
- Mentation, visual disturbances

- Libido, menstrual disorders
- Weakness, fatigue, changes in muscle activity
- Changes in respiration, pulse, and temperature; presence of dyspnea and palpitations
- Changes in elimination patterns (bowel and urinary)
- Frequent infections

Family History

- Endocrine disorders: acute or chronic
- Diabetes mellitus
- Thyroid disease
- Hypertension
- Obesity

Allergies

- Foods
- Medications
- Iodine

Patterns of Diabetes Mellitus Care

- Years disease present
- Insulin/hypoglycemic therapy
- Special dietary control

Activities of Daily Living (ADL)

- Abilities for self-care and/or ADL
- Ability to follow regimen for diabetes mellitus
- Special diet: diabetic, low calorie, or low fat
- Exercise requirements
- Homebound status

Psychosocial History

- Tobacco and alcohol use: daily and over period of years
- Personality traits
- Stress from occupation or chronic condition
- Adaptation to illness or chronic condition
- Cultural preferences in diet

Past Treatments and Diagnostic Procedures

- Medications (prescribed or OTC) taken for endocrine or other conditions
- Ultrasonograms, scans, x-ray studies of skull
- Laboratory tests for complete blood counts, glucose, thyroid function, and electrolytes
- Exposure to or treatment with radiation
- Surgery of any gland

■ Past or recent hospitalizations

Present History

Chief Complaint, Including Onset, Length of Time Present, and Severity

Signs and Symptoms

■ Weakness, fatigue, muscle weakness, twitching, spasms, numbness, tingling, cramping, tremors, wasting, reduced strength
■ Bone pain, aching
■ Nervousness, irritability, drowsiness, confusion
■ Libido changes
■ Anxiety, depression, apathy, syncope
■ Pruritis
■ Headache, malaise
■ Anorexia, nausea, vomiting
■ Polyuria, polydipsia

Knowledge of Disease and Planned Home Therapy

Present Treatments and Diagnostic Procedures

■ Diagnostic procedures and test results
■ Medications (oral, parenteral)
  ■ Insulin
  ■ Hypoglycemics
  ■ Steroids
  ■ Thyroid preparation
  ■ Male/female sex hormones

Physical Examination

Inspection

■ Vital signs, height, weight
■ Symmetry of extremities, edema (location, type, grade)
■ Skin color, turgor, dryness, oiliness, texture, edema, distribution of fat
■ Nail texture; hair amount, distribution, and texture
■ Moon face, protruding eyeballs, thickening of tongue, hoarseness, breath odor

Palpation

■ Decreased deep reflexes or absence of reflexes
■ Thyroid enlargement, hardness, nodules, or asymmetry (thyroid normally not palpable)

Hematologic System Assessment

Past History

Blood Disorders and Disorders of Blood-Forming Organs

- Anemias
- Leukemia, lymphoma
- Immune disorders
- Hemophilia
- Other blood dyscrasias
- Surgery (splenectomy)

Signs and Symptoms of Hematologic Diseases

- Weight loss
- Fatigue, weakness, pallor, shortness of breath
- Pain in bones or joints
- Bleeding from any site, bruising on body parts
- Enlarged nodes

Family History

- Hematologic disorders: acute or chronic
- Anemias
- Hemophilia
- Sickle cell trait
- Allergies
- Malignancies

Allergies

- Foods
- Medications
- Chemicals

Activities of Daily Living (ADL)

- Abilities for self-care and/or ADL
- Special diet: high iron or folic acid
- Homebound status

Psychosocial History

- Personality traits
- Lifestyle, including drug habits and sexual orientation
- Occupation and exposure to chemicals, lead, and other toxic agents or environmental pollutants
- Alcohol consumption: amount and duration

- Adaptation to illness or chronic condition

Past Treatments and Diagnostic Procedures

- Transfusions of blood or blood products and response
- Bone marrow transplant
- Medications (prescribed and OTC) taken for hematologic or other conditions
- Bone marrow puncture, scans, node biopsy
- Laboratory tests for complete blood count, platelets, reticulocytes, prothrombin time, and iron level
- Past or recent hospitalization
- Surgery of any kind

Present History

Chief Complaint, Including Onset and Length of Time Present

Signs and Symptoms

- Change in behavior, level of consciousness
- Fatigue, weakness, dizziness, headache, pallor, shortness of breath
- Pain in bones or joints, mouth, or tongue
- Anorexia, nausea, emaciation
- Night sweats
- Small or large hemorrhages on skin
- Bleeding from any site (prolonged or excessive)

Knowledge of Disease and Planned Home Therapy

Present Treatments and Diagnostic Procedures

- Laboratory and diagnostic tests and results
- Medications (oral, parenteral)
  - Antiinfectives
  - Antiinflammatories
  - Immunosuppressives
  - Antineoplastics
  - Tranquilizers
  - Antituberculins
  - Iron, folic acid
  - Vitamin B_{12}
  - Others

Physical Examination

Inspection

- Vital signs, height, weight
- Ecchymoses or petechiae
- Buccal cavity for edema, redness, bleeding, or ulceration
- Skin color, texture, pruritis
- General appearance for dehydration or cachexia

Palpation

- Size of liver and spleen
- Lymph nodes: enlargement, tenderness, movement, size, and consistency in neck, axilla, and inguinal areas
- Joint swelling

Musculoskeletal System Assessment

Past History

Muscle, Bone, and Joint Disorders

- Arthritis and type
- Bursitis
- Fractures
- Gout
- Low back syndrome
- Osteoporosis
- Paget's disease
- Ruptured disk
- Bone malignancy
- Neuromuscular disease
- Musculoskeletal surgery or injury (amputation, hip/knee replacement, laminectomy)

Signs and Symptoms of Musculoskeletal Disorders

- Pain or swelling in joints
- Muscle weakness, twitching, or deterioration
- Poor coordination or balance in walking or other movement
- Changes in range of motion (ROM) and activity and mobility
- Presence of cast or splint or use of traction for fracture or to provide support
- Paralysis
- Burning, numbness, and tingling in extremities
- Contracture(s), abnormal body alignment

■ Pathologic fractures

Family History

■ Joint or bone disorders: acute or chronic
■ Neurologic motor deficits
■ Neuromuscular disease
■ Musculoskeletal disease

Allergies

■ Foods
■ Medications
■ Chemicals

Activities of Daily Living (ADL)

■ Abilities for self-care and/or ADL
■ Use of aids for eating, toileting, dressing, and personal hygiene/care
■ Ability to use hands and fingers to grasp and hold objects
■ Ability to walk: energy and endurance and effect on joints
■ Special diet: low uric acid, high calcium, or low calorie
■ Homebound status

Psychosocial History

■ Tobacco, alcohol, and chemical consumption: daily and over period of years
■ Personality traits
■ Occupation and need for mobility and dexterity; proneness to accidents
■ Adaptation to disability or chronic illness

Past Treatments and Diagnostic Procedures

■ Medications (prescribed and OTC) taken for bone, muscle, or joint disease
■ Physical and occupational therapy and rehabilitation
■ Cold or heat applications
■ X-ray studies, scans, electromyogram, myelogram
■ Laboratory tests for electrolytes, uric acid, sedimentation rate, rheumatoid factor, complete blood count, and alkaline phosphatase
■ Use of TENS stimulator
■ Bone or joint surgery, use of cast or traction
■ Past or recent hospitalizations

Present History

Chief Complaint, Including Onset and Length of Time Present

Signs and Symptoms
- Pain in affected area
- Redness, swelling, or warmth in affected area
- Weakness, fatigue
- Loss of mobility, coordination or balance, or weight-bearing ability
- Limited ROM
- Loss of sensation in extremity
- Muscle spasms, reduced muscle strength and mass
- Diminished peripheral pulse in extremities, delayed capillary refill

Knowledge of Disease and Planned Home Therapy

Present Treatments and Diagnostic Procedures
- Laboratory and diagnostic tests and results
- Use of trapeze, cast, brace, traction, and aids for ADL
- Presence of limb prosthesis
- Bed rest, chair, amount of activity allowed
- Medications (oral)
  - Analgesics
  - Antirheumatics
  - Antiinflammatories (steroid and nonsteroid)
  - Muscle relaxants
  - Antibiotics
  - Stool softeners
  - Vitamin and mineral supplements (calcium and vitamin D)
  - Others

Physical Examination

Inspection
- Symmetry of legs and arms, shoulders, clavicles, scapulae, and musculature
- Full ROM of all joints; degree of motion
- Ability to sit, lie, get up, stand, and walk; posture
- Deformities or contractures, deviations, changes in contour
- Presence of scoliosis, kyphosis, lordosis, or hammer toe
- Gait, coordination, balance, endurance

- Body alignment in supine, prone, and side-lying positions
- Amputation
- Presence of enforced immobilization
- Skin of casted extremity or body part (pink, warm, dry with sensation present, peripheral pulse felt)
- Ability to move toes/fingers on casted part

Palpation

- Warmth and pain at joint(s) or injury
- Crepitus from joint motion
- Muscles for strength, mass, and tone
- Reflexes for presence
- Tenderness on pressure or movement
- Thickening, bony enlargement around joints

Renal/Urinary System Assessment

Past History

Kidney and Bladder Disorders

- Renal failure
- Pyelonephritis, glomerulonephritis
- Calculi
- Urinary tract infection
- Neurogenic bladder
- Prostatic hypertrophy
- Hypertension
- Kidney transplant
- Renal or bladder surgery

Signs and Symptoms of Renal/Urinary Disorders

- Pain in kidney or bladder area
- Urinary incontinence, bladder distention
- Retention, hesitancy, dribbling, urgency, frequency, burning, dysuria, nocturia
- Urine amount, color, sedimentation, hematuria, pus, mucus, clarity, and odor
- Polyuria, oliguria, anuria
- Weight gain
- Type and amount of fluid intake and output for 24 hours
- Edema, distention, fever, bruising, restlessness, insomnia
- Skin: dryness, itching, and poor turgor; dry lips and mucous membranes
- Mentation changes

Family History
- Renal or bladder disorders: acute or chronic
- Congenital or familial renal or urinary conditions
- Hypertension
- Connective tissue disorder
- Diabetes mellitus

Allergies
- Foods
- Medications

Activities of Daily Living (ADL)
- Abilities for self-care (toileting)
- Special diet: low in salt, potassium, calcium, or protein

Psychosocial History
- Tobacco, caffeine, and alcohol use: daily and over period of years
- Personality traits
- Sexually transmitted diseases
- Exposure to environmental or occupational nephrotoxic substance (heavy metals, carbon tetrachloride, phenols, pesticides)
- Adaptation to illness or chronic condition

Past Treatments and Diagnostic Procedures
- Presence of urinary diversion: type, care, and response
- Medications (prescribed and OTC) taken for renal/urinary or other conditions
- Ultrasonogram; scans; intravenous pyelogram; x-ray studies of kidney, ureter, and bladder; cystoscopy; kidney biopsy
- Laboratory tests for blood urea, nitrogen, creatinine, urinalysis, urine culture, and others
- Surgeries, trauma, or use of instruments in manipulation of tract during procedures
- Past or recent hospitalizations

Present History

Chief Complaint, Including Onset, Length of Time Present, Precipitating Factors, and Alleviating Factors if Relevant

Signs and Symptoms
- Pain

- Weight gain, edema
- Changes in urinary pattern
- Changes in urinary characteristics
- Anorexia, nausea, vomiting
- Thirst, dry skin, poor turgor
- Weakness, muscle cramping
- Pruritis, visual changes
- Fluid imbalance
- Electrolyte imbalance

Knowledge of Disease and Planned Home Therapy

Present Treatments and Diagnostic Procedures

- Diagnostic procedures and laboratory results
- Current fluid requirements and restrictions
- Use of urinary drainage devices or catheterizations
- Hemodialysis or peritoneal dialysis
- Dietary restrictions
- Medications (oral)
    - Analgesics
    - Diuretics
    - Antiinfectives
    - Steroids
    - Anticoagulants
    - Others

Physical Examination

Inspection

- Blood pressure elevation
- Skin color, pruritis, petechiae, ecchymoses, dryness, urate crystals
- Oral mucous membranes: dry, redness, or ulcerations
- Edema of hands, feet, sacral region, or legs; abdominal distention; neck vein distention
- Urinary output and characteristics with or without indwelling catheter
- Behavior changes in regard to alertness, confusion, cognitive ability, and level of consciousness
- Fruity or urine odor to breath, foul odor to urine
- Condition of urinary diversion site, dialysis shunt or abdominal site, or urinary catheter site

Palpation

- Size and movement of kidneys

- Pain in kidney or bladder area
- Bladder distention, abdominal distention

Percussion

- Dullness over bladder if distended

Integumentary System Assessment

Past History

Skin Disorders

- Dermatitis
- Acne
- Eczema
- Infestations, scabies, lice
- Infections of skin, nails, or scalp
- Skin malignancy
- Integumentary surgery (graft, cosmetic)

Signs and Symptoms of Integumentary Disorders

- Alopecia
- Dandruff
- Itching, breaks in skin
- Brittleness, ridging, redness, or swelling of nails and cuticles
- Tendency to have infections, herpes simplex
- Sensitivity to sun, soaps, deodorants, perfumes, and others
- Dryness, oiliness, excessive moisture, body odor
- Skin color changes
- Lumps or growths on the skin
- Bruising, delayed healing
- Ulcerations on extremity

Family History

- Integumentary disorders: acute or chronic
- Allergies, eczema

Allergies

- Foods
- Medications
- Cosmetics
- Environmental contacts

Activities of Daily Living (ADL)

- Pattern of bathing, with frequency and time; soap used; toothpaste, shaving cream, and razor used; and lotions and powders used
- Pattern of hair and nail care, with shampoo, rinse, and nail polish used; hair tint used; and cuticle trimming of toenails and fingernails
- Abilities for personal self-care
- Homebound status

Psychosocial History

- Personality traits, anxiety
- Effect on body image if dermatitis or scarring present
- Occupational exposure to irritants such as dyes, sprays, perfumes, and allergens
- Home environment exposure to allergens or irritants
- Adaptation to skin condition and effect on self-concept

Past Treatments and Diagnostic Procedures

- Desensitization therapy
- Medications (prescribed and OTC) taken for skin, hair, and nail conditions
- Skin biopsy
- Past or recent hospitalization

Present History

Chief Complaint, Including Onset and Length of Time Present

Signs and Symptoms

- Changes in skin color, eruptions, breaks, and precipitating factors
- Hair loss and precipitating factors
- Nail changes and precipitating factors
- Injury from burns, with degree of damage to skin and pain

Knowledge of Disease and Planned Home Therapy

Present Treatments and Diagnostic Procedures

- Laboratory and diagnostic tests and results
- Medications (oral, topical)
  - Antiinflammatories
  - Antipruritics
  - Antianxiety agents

- Antibiotics
- Antiacne agents
- Others

Physical Examination

Inspection

- Skin color for cyanosis, redness, jaundice, pallor, and pigmentation
- Bleeding, bruising
- Presence of striae, rashes, urticaria, or bites
- Skin dryness, oiliness, sweating, peeling, scaling, crusting
- Pruritis, odor, exudate, cleanliness
- Presence of edema, pain, breaks, or incision
- Lesions, lipomas, keloids, warts, nevi, with location and distribution
- Blisters, cellulitis, superficial infections
- Nail cleanliness; texture, thickness, and angle; ingrown nails or hangnails; presence of infection
- Hair cleanliness, quantity, texture, distribution, color, odors, brittleness, oiliness, or dryness; dandruff; baldness
- Scalp infestation, lesions

Palpation

- Skin temperature (hot or cool), texture (rough, bumpy, smooth, thin, thick)
- Skin turgor, elasticity, moisture, motility
- Tumors, cysts, or any elevation or lumps on skin or scalp
- Capillary return in nails and movement of nail plate when pressed

Reproductive System Assessment

FEMALE

Past History

Reproductive Disorders

- Sexually transmitted diseases
- Tubal pregnancy
- Abortions
- Pelvic inflammatory disease (PID)
- Infertility
- Menstrual disorders

- Endometriosis
- Breast, uterus, ovarian, or vaginal malignancy
- Surgery (mastectomy, hysterectomy)

Signs and Symptoms of Reproductive Organ Disorders

- Breast pain, tenderness, or discharge; change in nipple
- Dyspareunia
- Rashes or irritations of genitalia with pruritis
- Discharge from meatus or vagina
- Dysuria, urinary frequency, retention, incontinence
- Dysmenorrhea, amenorrhea

Family History

- Breast or reproductive malignancy (ovary, uterus)
- Reproductive disorders: acute or chronic

Allergies

- Scented feminine powders, pads, and tampons

Activities of Daily Living (ADL)

- Birth control use and effectiveness
- Breast self-examination and frequency, pap smear, mammogram
- Ability for toileting and genitalia hygiene
- Presence of indwelling catheter and ability for care
- Homebound status

Psychosocial History

- Personality traits
- Number of children, pregnancies
- Age at menarche; frequency, duration, and regularity of periods; amount of pain; bleeding between periods; last menstrual period
- Date or age of menopause, hot flashes, discharge, pain
- Intercourse frequency if active; satisfaction level
- Sexual orientation; multiple partners if appropriate
- Ability to carry out role function to satisfaction
- Adaptation to infertility or other chronic condition

Past Treatments and Diagnostic Procedures

- Intrauterine device, birth control implant
- Medications (prescribed and OTC) taken for gynecologic disorder

- Ultrasound, diagnostic dilatation and curettage, mammogram, laparoscopy, amniocentesis, breast or endometrial biopsy
- Laboratory tests for pregnancy, complete blood count, typing, and Rh factor
- Surgeries such as mastectomy (simple or radical), hysterectomy, salpingectomy, oophorectomy, cystocele or rectocele repair, or tubal sterilization
- Past or recent hospitalizations

Present History

Chief Complaint, Including Onset and Length of Time Present

Signs and Symptoms

- Abdominal pain, dysmenorrhea, amenorrhea
- Abnormal vaginal bleeding or discharge
- Genital pruritis, irritation
- Infertility
- Dyspareunia
- Dysuria

Knowledge of Disease and Planned Home Therapy

Present Treatments and Diagnostic Procedures

- Laboratory and diagnostic tests and results
- Use of birth control devices
- Radiation or chemotherapy
- Presence of urinary catheter
- Medications (oral, vaginal)
  - Hormones
  - Antibiotics
  - Antiinflammatories
  - Analgesics
  - Fertility therapy
  - Others

Physical Examination

Inspection (as appropriate)

- External genitalia for discharge, redness, swelling, ulcerations or lesions, or inflammation
- Bulging of vaginal walls
- Pediculosis pubis

- Cervical color, position, ulceration, bleeding, discharge, and masses
- Vaginal mucosa color, inflammation, ulcers, and masses
- Breast size, symmetry, contour, moles, dimpling, rash, edema, venous pattern, and color
- Nipple size, shape, discharge, rash, ulcers, and induration

Palpation

- Vaginal muscle tone, nodules, and tenderness
- Cervical position, shape, mobility, consistency, and tenderness
- Uterine size, shape, consistency, motility, tenderness, and masses
- Breast elasticity, fullness, tenderness, and nodosity
- Nipple elasticity, discharge with pressure
- Axillary nodes
- Masses in breasts: size, shape, location, consistency, motility, and tenderness

MALE

Past History

Reproductive Disorders

- Sexually transmitted diseases
- Hernia
- Prostatitis
- Hydrocele
- Epididymitis
- Prostatic hypertrophy
- Surgery (prostatectomy, penile implant, orchiectomy)

Signs and Symptoms of Reproductive Organ Disorders

- Pain in scrota, testes
- Discharge from penis
- Lesions on penis
- Impotence
- Urinary difficulty with urgency, frequency, or weak stream; difficulty starting or stopping; incontinence; inability to empty bladder

Family History

- Reproductive disorders: acute or chronic

Activities of Daily Living (ADL)

- Scrotal self-examination and frequency
- Ability for toileting and genitalia hygiene
- Presence of indwelling catheter and ability for care
- Homebound status

Psychosocial History

- Personality traits
- Intercourse frequency if active; satisfaction level
- Sexual orientation; multiple partners if appropriate
- Ability to carry out role function to satisfaction
- Effect of impotence on self-concept
- Adaptation to illness, impotence, infertility, or other chronic condition

Past Treatments and Diagnostic Procedures

- Penile device or implant
- Medications (prescribed and OTC) taken for reproductive disorders
- Cystoscopy, prostate biopsy
- Laboratory tests for urinary culture, complete blood count, and enzymes
- Surgeries such as vasectomy, prostatectomy, herniorrhaphy, orchiectomy, or penile implantation
- Past or recent hospitalizations

Present History

Chief Complaint, Including Onset and Length of Time Present

Signs and Symptoms

- Urinary abnormalities
- Pain in area
- Bleeding or discharge from penis
- Genital pruritis, irritation
- Penile lesions, ulcers, soreness

Knowledge of Disease and Planned Home Therapy

Present Treatments and Diagnostic Procedures

- Laboratory and diagnostic tests and results
- Use of aids/device for impotence
- Radiation or chemotherapy
- Presence of urinary catheter

- Medications (oral)
  - Analgesics
  - Antibiotics
  - Antispasmodics
  - Antiinflammatories
  - Hormones
  - Others

Physical Examination

Inspection

- Penis, meatus, and scrotum for ulcers, scars, rashes, nodules, discharge, or swelling
- Circumcision and cleanliness
- Pediculosis pubis
- Urethral meatus position
- Size and shape of penis for age
- Contour of scrota; testes in place
- Breast and nipple symmetry, lesions, drainage, and induration

Palpation

- Penile shaft for masses, tenderness, and induration
- Testes for size, shape, consistency, tenderness, and symmetry
- Prostate (rectal examination): softness, swelling, and tenderness
- Hernia (via inguinal canal)
- Breasts or nipples for masses, tenderness, or discharge on pressure

Eye, Ear, Nose, and Throat Assessment

Past History

Eye, Ear, Nose, and Throat Disorders

- Infections
- Glaucoma
- Cataracts
- Retinal detachment
- Tonsillitis
- Deviated septum, nasal polyps
- Allergic rhinitis
- Presbyopia, presbycusis
- Macular degeneration

■ Surgery or injury (tonsillectomy, enucleation, cataract, keratoplasty)

Signs and Symptoms of Eye, Ear, Nose, or Throat Disorders

■ Eye, ear, nose, or throat pain
■ Discharge from eye, ear, or nose
■ Multiple colds
■ Halitosis
■ Buzzing or roaring in the ears
■ Loss of equilibrium, vertigo
■ Headaches
■ Difficulty in swallowing
■ Runny or stuffy nose, epistaxis
■ Hoarseness
■ Changes in visual and auditory acuity

Family History

■ Eye, ear, nose, and throat disorders: acute or chronic
■ Allergies
  ■ Foods
  ■ Medications
  ■ Environmental pollutants
  ■ Animals
  ■ Chemicals
  ■ Other

Activities of Daily Living (ADL)

■ Effects of visual or auditory impairment
■ Use of glasses or contact lenses, eye prosthesis
■ Use of hearing aid, lip reading, signing
■ Loss of teeth and use of partial or full dentures
■ Changes in sense of smell or taste
■ Ability to perform self-care and care of glasses, contacts, prosthesis, dentures, or hearing aid; ability to instill eye drops
■ Response to hair sprays, noise levels, use of cotton swabs to clean ears, mouthwash
■ Homebound status

Psychosocial History

■ Effect of impairment on self-concept and occupation
■ Personality traits, anxiety or depression
■ Home environment exposure to allergens and irritants
■ Effects of age and emotions on impairment or disease
■ Adaptation to illness or impairment

Past Treatments and Diagnostic Procedures

- Densensitization therapy
- Medications (prescribed and OTC) taken for ear, eye, nose, or throat conditions or other conditions
- Last visit to dentist
- Date of most recent hearing or vision testing
- Laboratory tests for complete blood count and throat and nasal culture
- Skull x-ray studies, ocular procedures, laser procedure
- Surgeries such as tonsillectomy; cataract, corneal, or retinal surgery; stapedectomy; mastoidectomy; submucous resection; polypectomy
- Past or recent hospitalization

Present History

Chief Complaint, Including Onset and Length of Time Present

Signs and Symptoms

- Pain or soreness in area
- Onset, duration, precipitating factors if any
- Dysphagia, difficulty in chewing
- Discharge from eye, ear, nose, or throat
- Redness or swelling of eye, throat, or nasal mucosa
- Epistaxis
- Changes in sensory perception and acuity
- Temperature elevation
- Hoarseness, loss of voice

Knowledge of Disease and Planned Home Therapy

Present Treatments and Diagnostic Procedures

- Laboratory and diagnostic tests and results
- Nasal packing, eye covering and dressing
- Eye, ear, and throat irritations
- Medications (oral, drops, topical)
  - Analgesics
  - Antibiotics
  - Antiinflammatories
  - Antiglaucoma agents
  - Decongestants
  - Others

Physical Examination

Inspection

- Symmetry of eyes, lids, brows, and ears
- Lids: color, structure, edema, and lesions
- Conjunctival and scleral color; opacities; markings of iris
- Pupils: size, shape, equality, and reaction
- Intactness of extraocular movements
- Round, intact lacrimal glands; moisture or dryness of eyes
- External ears and auricles for lesions and deformities
- External ears and auricles for color, size, and position
- Canals and tympanic membranes, drainage
- Nose deformities, shape, symmetry, color, edema, drainage, bleeding, septal alignment
- Lips: color, dryness, cracking, edema, or ulcers
- Gums, buccal cavity, and throat: color, swelling, bleeding, or inflammation
- Tonsils (if present) for redness, swelling, or pus

Palpation

- Pinnae for firmness, masses, elasticity, and pain
- Structure of nose
- Tenderness in frontal or maxillary sinuses

Psychosocial Assessment*

Mental/Cognitive/Learning Assessment

Past History

- Educational level, educational achievements
- Attitude toward learning, ambition
- Difficulties in achieving educational or vocational goals
- Learning disabilities
- Interest in and willingness to learn about care and procedures
- Ability to listen and comprehend information given
- Ability to read and follow written instructions
- Vocabulary level and attention span
- Memory and ability to recall events
- Hearing, visual impairments
- English spoken or English as a second language

Present History

- Knowledge and understanding of illness and prognosis
- Cerebral function, including orientation, memory, recall, concentration, level of consciousness, and communication pattern
- Sensory function, including vision and hearing
- Physical ability, strength for self-care
- Ability to think rationally, make judgments, and problem solve
- Ability to express needs and maintain record of care and procedures

Psychiatric Assessment

Past History

- Psychiatric treatments, therapist
- Institution, including discharge dates
- Attitude toward treatments
- Medications prescribed, street or recreational drugs used
- Alcohol intake: amount and length of time
- Suicide potential and precipitating factors

*All assessments provided in this section are from Jaffe MS and Skidmore-Roth L: *Home health nursing care plans, ed. 2*, St. Louis, 1993, Mosby-Year Book, Inc.

- Family history of mental disorders
- Relationships with family members and feelings about family

Present History

- Personal appearance: hygiene, clothing, physical characteristics, posture, mannerisms, facial expression, and gestures
- Communication: tone, quality, flow, speed, use of associative looseness, flight of ideas, blocking, mutism, circumstantiality, word salad, and echolalia
- Mood, affect
- Orientation to time, place, and person
- Delusions, hallucinations, illusions
- Coping ability and skills
- Stressors present
- Presence of chronic anxiety, worry, depression, or insomnia
- Lives alone, isolation, support of significant others
- Lives with others but isolates self
- Participation in social interactions and activities

Advance Directives

- Awareness of Patient Self-Determination Act and its requirements and need for written information about advance directives
- Presence of an advance directive or form for health care
- Living will
- Durable power of attorney for health care
- Family understanding of and conflicts about client's directives
- Knowledge of rights of autonomy and consent to or refusal of care in home
- Location of the advance directive or a copy

Spiritual

- Religious beliefs and practices
- Feelings about a supreme being and how this view deals with illness
- Feelings about what will happen during illness
- Specific people helpful in religious life
- Religious symbols of importance (Bible, prayer, rosary, literature)

- Rituals of importance (communion, lighting Sabbath candles, Sacrament of the Sick)
- Religious restrictions (dietary laws, fasting, blood transfusion, medical treatment, birth control, abortion)
- Need for church attendance, priest, minister, or rabbi
- Identified spiritual leader

Occupational/Recreational Assessment

Past History
- Type of past employment
- Feelings about past employment
- Effects on health
- Reasons for leaving or changing vocation
- Presence of occupational hazards
- Hobbies and avocational activities

Present History
- Type of present employment/retirement
- Feelings about work/retirement
- Activity involved in work
- Effect of work environment on health (stress, chemicals, allergens)
- Plans for returning to work
- Housekeeping tasks (amount, kind, participation)
- Need for more education or wish for vocational retraining
- Type, frequency, and degree of participation in play and recreation
- Effect of illness on recreational interests/hobbies
- Alternative interests and activities while illness is present
- Need to change recreational activities permanently
- Adaptation to retirement and role changes

Functional Assessment*

General

- Homebound status, complete bed rest, activity restrictions
- Independence or dependence in self-care and activities of daily living and desire and willingness to perform and adapt to limitations (see Table 8 for the Index of Independence in Activities of Daily Living)
- Degree of disability or handicap
- Presence of artificial limb
- Rehabilitation therapy by physical and/or occupational therapist

Bathing/Grooming

- Ability to wash body (shower, tub bath, sponge bath)
- Use of aids to bathe (long handles for sponge, mitt on hand, bars in tub or shower, skid-proof tub, stool in tub or shower stall; wheelchair accessible facilities if needed)
- Ability to brush teeth and hair (brushing, soaking, comb, dryer)
- Use of aids to brush teeth and hair (long and built-up handles, extension handles, mounted dryer or brush with suction cup, squeeze bottles for shampoo and toothpaste)
- Ability to shave or apply makeup (electric or safety razor, makeup kit)
- Use of aids to shave or apply makeup (shaving cream, mirror mounted with suction cups, built-up handles, hanging mirror around neck)

Dressing/Undressing

- Type of clothing easy to put on and remove (loose fitting, elastic at waist, closures with zipper or Velcro, shoes with Velcro closures, wide openings to slip over head or slip on with front open)
- Ability to dress and undress (manage buttons and zippers,

*All assessments provided in this section are from Jaffe MS and Skid-more-Roth L: *Home health nursing care plans,* ed. 2, St. Louis, 1993, Mosby-Year Book, Inc.

tie laces, apply shoes and stockings)
- Use of aids for dressing (hooks, zippers, long handles for stockings and shoes)

Toileting

- Ability to use bathroom, commode, bedpan, or urinal
- Use of aids for toileting (grab bars, mounted toilet seat with side arms, tongs or mounting for toilet tissue)

Feeding

- Ability to feed self: partial or total assistance; ability to prepare meal
- Use of aids for eating (china and flatware with suction cups, flatware with swivel, extension handles on flatware, bumper guard on dishes, bib for droppings, cuff to hold utensils)
- Use of aids for drinking (grippers on cup or glass; large handles; long, bending straws; suction cups for cup or glass)

Mobility

- Ability to walk, sit, stand, or lie down; amount of assistance needed
- Use of aids for mobility and movement (wheelchair, walker, crutches, cane, brace, elevated chair, adjustable seat or ejector chair, footstool, trapeze, holding rails, mechanical lift), hospital bed (electric or semielectric)

Miscellaneous

- Book holder, tilted table, clipboard, holder for pencil, card or pad holder, mounts on chair for radio or books, remote control for electric appliances
- Cars with special modifications, use of vans or buses with wheelchair lift
- Magnifiers, large-print reading materials and telephone, amplifier on phone, special wiring for turning lights on or to alert client if deaf
- Automatic dialer and speaker phone attachment

Table 8   Index of Independence in Activities of Daily Living

The Index of Independence in Activities of Daily Living is based on an evaluation of the functional independence or dependence of clients in bathing, dressing, going to toilet, transferring, continence, and feeding. Specific definitions of functional independence and dependence appear below the index.

A— Independent in feeding, continence, transferring, going to toilet, dressing, and bathing.

B— Independent in all but one of these functions.

C— Independent in all but bathing and one additional function.

D— Independent in all but bathing, dressing, and one additional function.

E— Independent in all but bathing, dressing, going to toilet, and one additional function.

F— Independent in all but bathing, dressing, going to toilet, transferring, and one additional function.

G— Dependent in all six functions.

Other—Dependent in at least two functions, but not classifiable as C, D, E, or F.

Independence means without supervision, direction, or active personal assistance, except as specifically noted below. This is based on actual status and not on ability. A client who refuses to perform a function is considered as not performing the function, even though he or she is deemed able.

Bathing (Sponge, Shower, or Tub)

Independent: assistance only in bathing a single part (as back or disabled extremity) or bathes self completely
Dependent: assistance in bathing more than one part of body; assistance in getting in or out of tub or does not bathe self

Transfer

Independent: moves in and out of bed independently and moves in and out of chair independently (may or may not be using mechanical supports)
Dependent: assistance in moving in or out of bed and/or chair; does not perform one or more transfers

(Continued)

Table 8   Index of Independence in Activities of Daily Living (cont'd)

Dressing

Independent: gets clothes from closets and drawers; puts on clothes, outer garments, or braces; manages fasteners; act of tying shoes is excluded
Dependent: does not dress self or remains partly undressed

Going to toilet

Independent: gets to toilet; gets on and off toilet; arranges clothes; cleans organs of excretion (may manage own bedpan used at night only and may or may not be using mechanical supports)
Dependent: uses bedpan or commode or receives assistance in getting to and using toilet

Continence

Independent: urination and defecation entirely self-controlled
Dependent: partial or total incontinence in urination or defecation; partial or total control by enemas, catheters, or regulated use of urinals and/or bedpans

Feeding

Independent: gets food from plate or its equivalent into mouth (precutting of meat and preparation of food, such as buttering bread, are excluded from evaluation)
Dependent: assistance in act of feeding (see above); does not eat at all or parenteral feeding

Katz S et al.: *Studies of illness in the aged*, JAMA 185, September 21, 1963.

Environmental Assessment

Home Modifications*

- Call bell, water, tissues, wastebasket, and telephone within reach
- Space for equipment and supplies near client
- Space for storage of extra equipment and supplies
- Door wide enough to accommodate wheelchair or commode
- Laundry facilities for clothing, linens, and supplies
- Bathroom and commode within access for use
- Hot and cold running water or means to heat water
- Ramp or other access to home
- Room on first floor (if possible or if client is unable to use stairway) with window, ventilation, and temperature control
- Scales for weight in bathroom or near bed
- Hospital bed, trapeze connection
- Chair to assist client to standing position

Safety Factors*

- Client's feeling of safety in home
- Cleanliness of home, disorder, noise, waste disposal
- Safety bars and aids for ambulation and activities of daily living (ADL)
- Refrigeration for foods, medications, and supplies
- Proper lighting, arrangement of furniture, clear pathways
- Frayed or loose wiring or electrical connections, grounding of equipment
- Pathways dry and not slippery
- Side rails up or bed in low position if client using hospital bed
- Ability to perform ADL independently or amount of assistance needed
- Isolation or protective isolation procedures carried out
- Proper body alignment and positioning if client is on bed rest
- Use of restraints and precautions taken
- Presence of allergens, smoke, dust, animals, plants, or sprays
- Use of aids for ADL and to prevent falls

*From Jaffe MS and Skidmore-Roth L: *Home Health Nursing Care Plans,* ed. 2, St. Louis, 1993, Mosby-Year Book, Inc.

- Available emergency numbers to call
- Proper cleansing and disinfection of reusable supplies
- Proper administration of medications and use of aids to ensure accuracy
- Proper handwashing procedure when required
- Presence of indoor plumbing versus drawn water and adequate storage for water
- Woodstove/kerosene heater safety and use and ability to fuel fire

Accessibility Checklist for the Home[*]

Outside/Approach
- Slope at entrance
- Parking near entrance
- Dimensions of walkway
- Connection of walkway to other surfaces (platforms, ramps)
- Surface nonskid

Ramps/Stairs
- Slope
- Dimensions
- Surface nonskid
- Handrails (height, side)
- Clearance at bottom
- Landing dimensions
- Edge protection (ramps)

Entrances
- Number
- Dimensions

Kitchen
- Doorway
- Door swings out/in to kitchen
- Counters
- Cupboards
- Sink
- Adequate lighting
- Outlets
- Controls for stove (front, back)

*From Bronstein KS, Popovich JM, and Stewart-Amidei C: *Promoting stroke recovery: A research-based approach for nurses*, St. Louis, 1991, Mosby-Year Book, Inc.

- Hot water pipes covered
- Water temperature regulated

Bathroom

- Doorway
- Door swings out/in to bathroom
- Commode
- Grab bars
- Space next to commode for w/c
- Bathtub
- Space next to tub for w/c
- Shower/tub faucets
- Shower
- Threshold into shower
- Sink
- Hot water pipes covered
- Water temperature regulated

Miscellaneous

- Telephones (location, number)
- Smoke detectors (location)
- Fire extinguisher (location)
- Flooring (type)
- Extension cords
- Throw rugs

Family Assessment*

Past and Present Physical History

- Chronic illness of family members
- Functional abilities or disabilities
- Health practices
- Types of practitioners used
- Medications taken by family members
- Energy levels of family members
- Physical strength and ability to perform procedures

Past and Present Psychosocial History

Emotional Status/Mental Abilities

- Changes in family life caused by client needs
- Willingness to perform procedures and care for client
- Support of client by member most likely to become caretaker
- Family attitude toward illness or disability
- Ability of family members to adapt
- Ability of family to set goals and problem solve
- Decision maker in the family
- Family stressors and ability to cope
- Relationship of client and family members
- Family arguments, separations, divorces

Psychiatric Disorders

- Chronic anxiety in family
- Depression of family member
- Behavior disorder of family member
- General mental health of family
- Presence of alcoholism, family violence, suicides, or drug abuse

Cultural Influences

- Spiritual beliefs
- Language barriers, English as second language
- Beliefs regarding health care and health professionals
- General values and ethnic identity of family

*All assessments provided in this section are from Jaffe MS and Skidmore-Roth L: *Home health nursing care plans, ed. 2*, St. Louis, 1993, Mosby-Year Book, Inc.

Economic Assessment*

Financial Resources

- Ability to perform financial responsibilities and handle money
- Occupation; effect of illness on work and ability to continue with same occupation
- Retirement income/effect of illness on limited income
- Ability to purchase or rent equipment, supplies, and services used in the home
- Possible number of home visits and cost
- Programs available to assist
  - Foundations
  - Churches
  - Voluntary agencies and support groups
  - National associations
  - Government grants
- Qualification for Medicaid
- Third-party payers
  - Medicare, CHAMPUS
  - Private insurance
  - Veterans administration
  - Public aid

Resources For Equipment and Supplies

- Pharmacy and supply companies
- Home health agencies
- Home infusion and supply companies
- Durable equipment companies (purchase or rental)
- Medical supplies companies (disposable and reusable)
- Community organizations that offer medical supplies and financial assistance

*All assessments provided in this section are from Jaffe MS and Skidmore-Roth L: *Home health nursing care plans, ed. 2*, St. Louis, 1993, Mosby-Year Book, Inc.

Tools for Assessment

Because so much variety exists in home environments in home health nursing, additional assessment tools and checklists are included here. The extent to which the items in each of the following checklists will be useful varies, of course, depending on each client's needs. In addition, the extent of the client's collaboration in these evaluations will also depend on each client's condition; the home health nurse should modify use of these checklists accordingly.

Home Assessment Checklist*

General Household

1. Is there good lighting available, especially around stairwells?
2. Are there handrails (which can be easily grasped) on both sides of the staircases, designed to indicate when top and bottom steps have been reached?
3. Are top and bottom steps painted in easily seen colors? Are nonskid treads used?
4. Are the edges of rugs tacked down? (Suggest the use of wall-to-wall carpeting.)
5. Is a telephone present? Does the telephone have a dial that is easily readable? Are emergency numbers written in large print and kept near the telephone?
6. Are electrical cords, footstools, and other low-lying objects kept out of walkways?
7. Are electrical cords in good condition?
8. Is furniture arranged to allow for free movement in heavily traveled areas?
9. Is furniture sturdy enough to give support?
10. Is furniture designed to accommodate easy transfers on and off?
11. Is the temperature of the home within a comfortable range?
12. If fireplaces or other heating devices are present, do they have protective screens?
13. Are smoke detectors present (especially in the kitchen and bedroom)?
14. Are rapidly closing doors eliminated?
15. Are there alternative exits from the house?

*From Tideiksaar R: New York, 1983, Ritter Department of Geriatrics and Adult Development, The Mount Sinai Medical Center.

16. Are basements and attics easy to get to, well lighted, and well ventilated?
17. Are slippers and shoes in good repair? Do they fit properly and have nonskid soles?

Kitchen

18. Are there loose extension cords, small sliding rugs, or slippery linoleum tiles present? (Suggest the use of rubber-backed, nonskid rugs and nonskid floor wax.)
19. Is the cooking stove gas or electric?
20. Are there large, easily readable dials present on the stove or other appliances, with the "on" and "off" positions clearly marked?
21. Are refrigerators in good working order? Are refrigerators placed on 18-inch platforms to avoid bending over?
22. Are spaces for food storage adequate? Are shelves at eye level and easily reachable?
23. Is a sturdy stepladder present for reaching?
24. Are electrical circuits overloaded with too many appliances?
25. Are electrical appliances disconnected when not in use?
26. Are sharp objects (such as carving knives) kept in special holders?
27. Are cleaning fluids, polishes, bleaches, detergents, and all poisons stored separately and clearly marked?
28. Are kitchen chairs sturdy, with arm rests and high backs?
29. Is stove free from flammable objects?
30. Are pot holders available for removing pots and pans from the stove?
31. Is baking soda available in case of fire?

Bathroom

32. Are there grab bars in the bath, in the shower, and around the toilet?
33. Are toilet seats high enough to get on and off without difficulty?
34. Can the bathroom door be easily closed to ensure privacy? (Avoid locks.)
35. Are bathroom doorways wide enough for easy wheelchair and walker access?
36. Are there nonskid rubber mats in the bath, in the shower, and on the floor?
37. Is there good lighting in the area of the medicine cabinet?

38. Are internal and external medications stored separately? and safely (especially important with young children or grandchildren present in the house)?
39. Do medication containers have childproof tops? Are they labeled in large print? Is a magnifying glass present for reading medication instructions?
40. Have all outdated medications been discarded?
41. Are there any medications (both prescription and OTC) that could cause adverse side effects or drug-drug interactions that the client is unaware of?
42. Can the water temperature be easily regulated?
43. Are electrical cords, outlets, and appliances a safe distance from the tub?
44. Are razor blades kept in a safe place?
45. Is a first aid kit available?

Bedroom

46. Is there adequate lighting from the bedside to the bathroom?
47. Are lights easily accessible? (If not, suggest keeping a flashlight by the bedside or using a flashlight for entry into dark rooms if light switch is not within easy reach.)
48. Are beds in good repair?
49. Are beds at the proper height to allow for easy transfer on and off without difficulty?
50. Do bedroom rugs have nonskid rubber backings?

Table 9   Assessment of Potential Risks for Accidents in the Home

- Activities of daily living (level of function)
- Cognition, emotional state (memory, depression)
- Clinical findings (health history)
- Incontinence
- Drugs (complete inventory)
- Eyes, ears, environment (sensory deficits)
- Neurologic deficits (gait, balance)
- Travel history (driving ability)
- Social history (alcohol, drug)

Escher JE, O'Dell C, and Gambert SR: Typical geriatric accidents and how to prevent them, *Geriatric* 44:57, 1989. Reprinted with permission.

Activities of Daily Living

The assessment of the client's ability to perform the activities of daily living provides the nurse with data to determine the client's self-care ability. The following tool may be used to plan the assistance given to the client to regain a maximum level of independence, and to plan for support services. Both basic activities of daily living and instrumental activities of daily living are included.*

Activities of Daily Living Assessment

I. Introduction
- A. Definition: Activities of daily living are those which a person performs on his or her own behalf in maintaining life, health, and well-being.
- B. Nursing assessment of client needs and functional abilities:
  1. Ability to communicate verbally and nonverbally
  2. Desire to engage in self-assessment and self-care
  3. Medical history relevant to disability and preexisting health status
  4. Social history
  5. Home responsibilities
  6. Home accessibility
  7. Education
  8. Vocational status
  9. Avocational testing
  10. Transportation issues
  11. Endurance and level of fatigue

II. Evaluation of activities of daily living
- A. Assess client's status using predetermined indicators and project discharge goals with evaluation of ADL:
  1. Use of assistive devices
  2. Ability to secure own equipment
  3. Toileting/cleansing
  4. Bathing (washing, drying)
  5. Care of teeth (brushing; denture care, including oral placement/removal and storage)
  6. Hair care (shampooing, brushing, combing)
  7. Skin care
  8. Grooming (social/psychological additions to general

*Mumma CM, editor: *Rehabilitation nursing concepts and practice: A core curriculum, ed. 2,* Skokie, Il., 1987, Rehabilitation Nursing Foundation.

appearance/self-image enhancement)
9. Dressing/undressing, upper and lower extremities
10. Eating (preparing meals and feeding self)
11. Personal care clean-up activities
12. Social/psychological activities
13. Kitchen tasks
14. Homemaking tasks
15. Child care
16. Community skills
17. Communication skills
18. Recreational activities
19. Sexual activity/function

B. Review findings of other team members.

III. Designed program to increase self-care abilities
  A. Program should include:
    1. Evaluation of client's current functional status and actual and potential problems
    2. Precautions to be exercised in view of medical status
    3. Client and family interactions and determination of primary caregiver
    4. Discharge plans and particular needs of client
    5. Treatment plan established with physician, therapist, client, family, nurse, and other team members

  B. Evaluate factors contributing to inability to perform activities of daily living:
    1. Situational or environmental factors (inaccessibility, sensory overload, etc.)
    2. Complexity of task and sequencing
    3. Impaired ability to focus attention on task
    4. Primary or secondary illnesses, disabilities, or deficits
    5. Visual neglect
    6. Impaired balance
    7. Impaired endurance, low activity tolerance due to fatigue
    8. Sensation deficit
    9. Coordination deficit
    10. Perceptual deficit
    11. Impaired judgment
    12. Impaired memory
    13. Communication deficit
    14. Apraxia
    15. Spasticity
    16. Contracture
    17. Pain

18. Paralysis
19. Paresis
20. Lack of one or more extremity(ies)
21. Visual impairment
22. Auditory impairment
23. Mobility deficit
24. Learning impairments
25. Psychological impairment
    a. Loss, grief, depression
    b. Self-image deficit
    c. Motivation (role in self-initiation of care tasks)
C. Specific elements to consider in activities of daily living training:
   1. Feeding
      a. Utensil, cup, and plate management and napkin use
      b. Tidiness/organization
      c. Awareness of swallowing, chewing, or pocketing problems
      d. Ability to handle different foot consistencies, e.g., finger foods vs. soups
      e. Mouth care after eating
   2. Bathing
      a. Assembling of items and appropriate equipment
      b. Management of caps, lids, sprays, etc.
      c. Facial cleansers and cosmetic application
      d. Shaving foam or soap application vs. electric razor
      e. Shaving face, underarms, and/or legs
      f. Hair care
      g. Deodorant application
      h. Tooth/denture care
      i. Nail care
      j. Replacement of care items
      k. Location of bath facilities in hospital and home
      l. Transfer ability to bathtub or shower
   3. Dressing
      a. Selection of clothing
      b. Assembling of clothing
      c. Application of underwear
      d. Management of fasteners
      e. Application of trousers/slacks and belt or suspenders
      f. Management of buckles and zippers
      g. Application of pullover tops

       h. Application of shirt, jacket, dress (front opening), or tie

       i. Management of buttons

       j. Application of socks or stockings

       k. Application of shoes, tying laces

       l. Location of dressing activities: bed, sitting, or standing

       m. Ability to care for and apply glasses, contact lenses, or hearing aid

4. Toileting and elimination management
   a. Transfer ability
   b. Clothing management
   c. Cognitive function
   d. Bowel and bladder control
   e. External devices: assembly, application, removal, and care of equipment
   f. Suppository insertion (include preparation of suppository and cleaning of insertion device if used)
   g. Post-toileting hygiene
   h. Timing of bowel program (morning or evening)
   i. Employment/school/home/environmental considerations
   j. Colostomy or ileal conduit care
   k. Performance of bladder management programs
   l. Accident management

Mental Status Assessment

I. General Appearance

Underweight   Overweight   Emaciated
Clean   Unkempt   Needs bath
Clothing appropriate to season/occasion
Peculiarity of dress/cosmetics
Explain and describe:

II. Motor Status

Posture: Erect   Stooped   Slouched
Muscular twitching   Grimacing   Posturing
Gait coordinated   Gait unsteady   Gait stiff
Shuffling   Other
Explain and describe:

_____
_____
_____

III. *Activity*

WNL Seizures   Lethargic   Purposeful
Disorganized activity   Restless at night   Bedridden
Explain and describe:

_____
_____
_____

IV. *Facial Expression*

Alert   Tense   Sad   Crying   Happy   Angry   Flat
Explain and describe:

_____
_____
_____

V. *Mood*

Angry   Depressed   Sad   Calm   Happy
Agitated   Labile   Other
Explain and describe:

_____
_____
_____

VI. *Environment*

Interest in family   Friends   Social activities
Environment

VII. *Orientation*

Oriented to: Time   Place   Person
Preoccupied   Distractable
Immediate memory   Recent memory   Distant memory
Complete disorientation

VIII. *Thought Processes*

Able to complete sentences   Jumps from topic to topic
Spontaneous   Mute   Logical   Illogical
Loose associations   Meaningless repetition of words
Decreased concentration ability   Mistakes in judgment

IX. *Thought Content*

Obsessions: Explain and describe:

_____

_____
_____

Compulsions: Explain and describe:

_____
_____
_____

Delusions: Explain and describe:

_____
_____
_____

X. Danger Assessment

Suicidal thoughts   Suicidal plans
Recent suicidal gesture and/or attempt

XI. Insight

Aware of present impairment?_____
What makes you think so?

_____
_____
_____

Aware of treatment need?_____
What makes you think so?

_____
_____
_____

Hogstel MO: *Clinical manual of gerontological nursing*, St. Louis, 1992, Mosby-Year Book, Inc.

General Considerations in Caring for Clients at Home

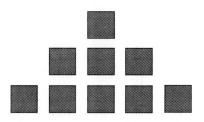

Nutrition

The Importance of Monitoring Diet in the Home Care Client

Nutrition is particularly important for homebound clients, whose general health is already compromised in some way. In addition, many clients seen in the home setting have special dietary needs, such as diabetics. Even something as ordinary as age group greatly affects one's health profile. For instance, the leading cause of death in middle age is heart disease, followed by malignant neoplasms, including colorectal cancer. Minimizing risks for both of these involves monitoring of diet, particularly high-fat, low-fiber diets (Beare & Myers, 1994).

In old age, these concerns are increased. Although older adults require fewer calories, they need greater amounts of trace elements and vitamins. Changes associated with aging may compound nutritional problems causing malnutrition. Milk and dairy products are an excellent source of protein and calcium for the older adult. However, many people have lactose intolerance. During nutritional counseling, keep in mind that a genetic predisposition toward lactose intolerance occurs in Asians, Native Americans, Eskimos, and other ethnic groups in which milk is not a traditional food.

Socioeconomic factors also play a role in nutrition. A limited income and a lack of interest in, or energy for, food preparation can promote a diet high in carbohydrates but limited in protein, fresh vegetables, and fruit. Psychosocial factors that may increase nutritional risk include living alone, loneliness, forgetfulness, or intentional starvation as a way of suicide. Mechanical high-risk factors are dental changes (loss of teeth, ill-fitting dentures), decreased strength and mobility, diminished vision, or polypharmacy. Diet guidelines to reduce costs can be included, offering teaching in terms of less expensive foods that still meet requirements for good nutrition (e.g., substituting vegetable proteins for meat) (Beare & Myers, 1994). The Food Guide Pyramid (USDA, 1992) is a useful tool for teaching clients about proper nutrition (see Figure 1).

The following assessment guide and tables can help the home health nurse recognize nutritional deficits or needs and formulate interventions to improve nutritional status.

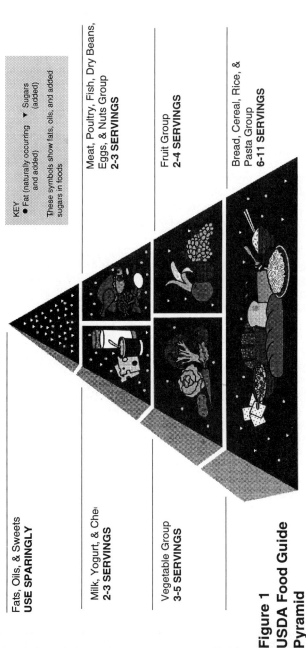

KEY
● Fat (naturally occurring   ▼ Sugars
  and added)   (added)

These symbols show fats, oils, and added sugars in foods

Meat, Poultry, Fish, Dry Beans, Eggs, & Nuts Group
2-3 SERVINGS

Fruit Group
2-4 SERVINGS

Bread, Cereal, Rice, & Pasta Group
6-11 SERVINGS

Fats, Oils, & Sweets
USE SPARINGLY

Milk, Yogurt, & Cheese
2-3 SERVINGS

Vegetable Group
3-5 SERVINGS

Figure 1
USDA Food Guide Pyramid

US Department of Agriculture: USDA food guide pyramid, USDA Human Nutrition Information Pub No 249, Washington, DC, 1992, US Government Printing Office.

Nutritional History Guidelines for Home Care Patients

Client name _____

Marital status _____

Age _____   Family or Significant Others

Gender _____   _____

                        _____

                        _____

                        _____

Primary medical diagnosis _____

Height _____   Weight _____

Recent weight change (note amount, time period, and
   cause) _____

Frame (small, medium, large) _____

Allergies (food or drug) _____

Smoking (packs per day)_____

Medications   _____   _____

                  _____   _____

Describe dosage schedule for medications, that is, are they
taken with meals or on an empty stomach? _____

Food preferences _____

_____

_____

Food intolerences or restrictions _____

_____

_____

Therapeutic diet or nutritional support prescription

_____

_____

_____

                                  (Continued)

Nutritional History Guidelines for Home Care Patients (cont'd)

What do the client or family find to be the easiest and most difficult parts of the therapeutic diet or nutritional support plan? _____
_____
_____

What, if anything, would the client or family like to change about the therapeutic diet or nutritional support plan?

_____
_____
_____

Usual daily dietary intake (including fluids)

_____
_____

Availability of foodstuffs:
Who does the shopping?_____
Where is shopping done? _____

Are there transportation problems with regard to shopping?_____

Is client limited by seasonal availability of foods? (Explain)
_____
_____

Financial concerns regarding diet _____
Cultural/religious concerns _____
What is the meaning of food to this family (e.g., social or sustenance only)?
_____
_____

Food storage_____
Refrigeration_____
Hygiene _____

(Continued)

Nutritional History Guidelines for Home Care Patients (cont'd)

Food preparation _____

Electricity, gas _____

Functioning stove, oven _____

Sufficient utensils _____

Who prepares the food? _____

Who makes food decisions?_____

Health problems (describe in terms of onset, chronology, quality, associated factors, aggravating factors, alleviating factors, how the problem is managed, and whether the intervention is effective) _____

_____

_____

Indigestion (pre- or post-prandial) _____

Dysphagia _____

Difficulty chewing _____

Diabetes _____

Cardiovascular disease _____

Hypertension _____

Condition of teeth/gums _____

Dentures (full, partial) _____

Sebastian T: *Nutrition in home care*. In Martinson I and Widmer J, editors: *Home health care nursing*, Philadelphia, 1989, WB Saunders Co.

Table 10   Physical Abnormalities in Nutritional Depletion

Location	Signs	Deficiencies
Hair	Alopecia	Protein-calorie
	Brittleness	Protein-calorie
	Dryness	Zinc
	Easy pluckability	Vitamins E and A
Head	Temporal wasting	Protein-calorie
	Soft spot that does not harden	Vitamin D
Eyes	Pale conjunctiva	Iron, folate, vitamin B_{12}
	Bitot's spots in children	Vitamin A
	Conjunctival xerosis	Vitamin A
Lips	Cracked, red, flaky corners	Riboflavin, niacin, iron, pyridoxine
Tongue	Edema	Folate, niacin
	Smooth tongue; atrophied taste buds	Riboflavin, iron, vitamin B_{12}
Gums	Pale	Iron
	Bleeding	Vitamins K and C
	Inflamed; sores	Vitamin C
Nails	Spooning	Iron
	Transverse lines; ridges	Protein-calorie

Turner J, McDonald G, and Larter N: *Handbook of pediatric and adult respiratory home care*, St. Louis, 1994, Mosby-Year Book, Inc.

Table 11   Common Laboratory Measures of Nutritional Status

Test	Normal Value	Comments
Serum albumin	3.5-5.5 g/dl	Low in malnutrition; most important test for protein-calorie deficiency; also reduced in liver disease
Creatinine height index	See comments	Measure of skeletal protein; requires 24-hr urine specimen; helpful when weight fluctuations caused by fluid loss or nutrition confuse clinical picture; most useful to monitor patient changes in muscle mass rather than comparison with any "normal" values
Total lympho-cyte count	1500-4000/µl	Measure of cellular immunity; low in diseases affecting cellular immunity such as HIV infection; low in protein-calorie deficiency
Serum transferrin	200-400 mg/dl	Serum globulin that binds and transports iron; low in malnutrition
Serum vitamin A	300-650 µg/L	Fat-soluble vitamins poorly absorbed in cystic fibrosis; water-soluble supplements often required; dose based on serum level
Serum vitamin E	5-20 µg/L	

Turner J, McDonald G, and Larter N: *Handbook of pediatric and adult respiratory home care*, St. Louis, 1994, Mosby-Year Book, Inc.

Table 12   Interventions for Problems Affecting Dietary Intake

Symptom	Approach for Client
Anorexia	Check with physician about possible adjustments in medications that may cause anorexia, such as theophylline and antibiotics.
	Try to eat even if appetite is poor because appetite usually improves with improved nutritional status.
	Try a glass of wine 1/2 hr before meals.
	Prepare aromatic foods such as fried onions or fresh baked bread.
	Have high-calorie foods readily available for snacks.
	Have bedtime snacks.
	Rely on favorite foods.
	Avoid huge portions of food, which may only overwhelm the patient.
	Eat small portions of food more frequently.
	Serve attractive meals.
	Make the meal an enjoyable event.
	Exercise 2 hrs after a meal.
	Rely on calorie-dense foods.
Early satiety	Eat high-calorie foods first.
	Limit liquids until the end of the meal or drink fluids between meals.
	Eat small amounts often.
Dyspnea	Rest before meal.
	Use bronchodilators or a caffeine drink 1/2 to 1 hr before meals.
	Implement secretion clearance strategies, if indicated, at least 1 hr before a meal to allow for rest before eating. A hot drink may

(Continued)

Table 12 Interventions for Problems Affecting Dietary Intake (cont'd)

Symptom	Approach for Client
	facilitate secretion clearance.
	Eat in a leisurely manner. Try soft music and a pleasant atmosphere. Practice relaxation techniques before eating to reduce anxiety and wheezing.
	Eat in a sitting position with the feet and elbows supported (tripod position).
	If dyspnea increases during the meal, rest for a short period while using pursed lip breathing until breathlessness subsides. Use pursed lip breathing between bites if breathlessness is severe.
	Use oxygen with meals if prescribed. Evaluate oxygen desaturation with meals with pulse oximeter and adjust flow rate of oxygen if necessary.
	Consider possible effect of high CHO intake on CO_2 production for patients who retain CO_2, and alter diet if indicated.
Fatigue	Prepare meals several hours before eating, then rest to conserve energy for meal.
	Prepare large amounts of food, then package food into serving sizes and freeze for later use.
	Use easy-to-prepare meals such as frozen or canned foods when tired.
	Use community agency meals such as Meals on Wheels.
	Give toddlers and preschool age children finger foods that are easy to chew so that they can pace their meal.
	Eat slowly and use foods that are easy to

(Continued)

Table 12   Interventions for Problems Affecting Dietary Intake (cont'd)

Symptom	Approach for Client
	chew and digest.
	Use tripod position.
	Infants with marginal sucking musculature should be fed with a soft pliable nipple, preferably with a cross-cut opening.
Depression	Make meals a pleasant experience.
	Encourage exercise.
	Encourage socialization.
	Seek treatment if depression is significant.
Anxiety	Make meals enjoyable.
	Avoid stressful discussions during meals.
	Practice relaxation before meal.
	Rest before meal.
	Watch favorite TV show while eating.
	Refer client for treatment if anxiety is significant.
Taste changes	Eat foods that taste good.
	Keep mouth moist to improve taste bud sensitivity.
	Suck on a sour candy or eat a pickle 1/2 hr before meal to stimulate taste.
	Keep nostrils clear so that sense of smell is enhanced.
	Clean teeth or dentures before meals.
Dry mouth	Consume enough fluids to prevent dehydration.
	Adjust medication schedule to limit dry mouth before meals.
	Suck on a sour candy or eat a pickle 1/2 hr before meal to stimulate salivation.

(Continued)

Table 12   Interventions for Problems Affecting Dietary Intake (cont'd)

Symptom	Approach for Client
	Humidify oxygen if flow rate is over 4 L/min.
Bloating	Eat small, frequent meals and stop eating when uncomfortable.
	Avoid rushed meals and relax before eating.
	Use controlled pursed lip breathing to prevent air swallowing.
	Prevent constipation.
	Avoid gas-forming foods that cause bloating.
	Position infant so that esophagus is higher than stomach during feeding.
	Most bottle feedings should take between 10 and 20 min.
Food aversion	Avoid foods that are disliked.
	Substitute different types of food that are high in calories.
	Do not mix disliked food into other foods.
Nausea/ vomiting	Check with physician about adjusting medications if indicated.
	Avoid foods that are unappetizing and highly spiced.
	Seek medical advice for other possible causes.
Diarrhea	Avoid hypertonic liquids.
	Avoid highly spiced foods.
	Seek medical advice.
Constipation	Implement a regular exercise program.
	Increase dietary fiber.

(Continued)

Table 12   Interventions for Problems Affecting Dietary Intake (cont'd)

Symptom	Approach for Client
	Ask physician about stool softeners.
Chewing problems	Facilitate proper dental care. Refit dentures if loose. Eat soft foods or liquids.
No social-ization	Participate in community center meal programs. Encourage asking friend to lunch or dinner. If eating alone, make the occasion enjoyable by watching favorite TV program or reading.
No meal preparation facilities	Refer to community meal facility or arrange home delivery of meals. Plan meals that are easily prepared with available facilities.
No support system	Arrange for grocery delivery. Arrange for someone to prepare meals. Arrange for community meal delivery. Evaluate for alternative living site.
Financial constraints	Refer for financial assistance through food stamp program, community meal assistance, or other program. Discuss inexpensive but nutritious foods and cost-saving measures such as bulk food purchases and food banks.

Turner J, McDonald G, and Larter N: *Handbook of pediatric and adult respiratory home care*, St. Louis, 1994, Mosby-Year Book, Inc.

Table 13   Enteral Nutritional Supplementation

Type	Form	Indications	Protein (%)	Caloric content Fat (%)	CHO (%)	Density (%) (Kcal/ml)
Complete formulations						
High density (e.g., Ensure, Sustacal, Instant Breakfast*)	Liquid	When balanced diet in liquid form required Replaces or supplements solid food	10-16	32-40	45-53	1.5-2.0
Isotonic (e.g., Isocal)	Liquid	Less sweet and isosmotic, often used for cancer patients	14-15	31-40	45-55	1-2.0
Modular diets (polycose)	Powder	When increased amounts of a specific nutrient required	—	—	100	(8 Kcal/ teaspoon)

* A good food supplement that is the least expensive of the formulations.

Turner J, McDonald G, and Larter N: *Handbook of pediatric and adult respiratory home care*, St. Louis, 1994, Mosby-Year Book, Inc.

Recommendations for the Diabetic Diet

Calories	To achieve or maintain desirable body weight
Carbohydrate	55% to 60% of total calories
	Replace low fiber with high fiber
Protein	12% to 20% of total calories
	0.8 g/kg of body weight
	Decrease with risk for or presence of nephropathy
Fat	< 30% of total calories
	Replace saturated fat with unsaturated
Cholesterol	< 300 mg/day
Fiber	Up to 40 g/day
	25 g/1000 Kcal daily for those on low-calorie diets
Sodium	≤ to 3000 mg/day
	Reduced in those with hypertension

Adapted from American Diabetes Association: Nutritional recommendations for individuals with diabetes mellitus, 1986, *Diabetes Care* 10, 1987, p. 126.

Maintaining and Improving Mobility

Mobility refers to a person's *ability* to move about freely, and immobility refers to the *inability* to move about freely. Mobility and immobility are best understood as the endpoints of a continuum, with many degrees of partial immobility in between. Some clients move back and forth on the mobility-immobility continuum, but for other clients, immobility is absolute and continues for an indefinite period.

When there is an alteration in mobility, each body system is at risk for impairment. The severity of the impairment depends on the client's age and overall health and the degree of immobility experienced. For example, elderly clients with chronic illnesses develop pronounced effects of immobility more quickly than do younger clients.

Changes in a client's mobility can result from various health problems. Examples of medical conditions that can alter mobility are musculoskeletal conditions such as fractured extremities or muscle sprains, neurologic conditions such as spinal cord trauma, degenerative neurologic conditions such as myasthenia gravis, and head injuries. Some clients may not actually be immobilized by an injury or musculoskeletal problem but are prescribed bed rest or restricted ambulation for therapeutic reasons, for example, for a cardiovascular condition or infectious problem.

Regardless of whether the cause of immobility is permanent or temporary, the immobilized client must receive some type of exercise to prevent excessive muscle atrophy and joint contractures. The total amount of activity required to prevent physical disuse syndrome is only about 2 hours for every 24-hour period, but this activity must be scheduled throughout the day to prevent the client from remaining inactive for long periods.

Exercises done in bed can help promote both joint mobility and muscle strength. Exercise prevents some of the complications of immobility and helps prepare a client for ambulation.

Range-of-motion (ROM) exercises put each joint through as full a range of motion as possible without causing discomfort. ROM exercises may be *active, passive,* or *active-assisted.* They are *active* if the client is able to perform the exercises independently and *passive* if the exercises are performed for the client by someone else. *Active-assisted* exercises are done by a client with some assistance. A client who is weak or partially paralyzed may be able to move a limb partially through its range of motion. In this case the nurse can help the client perform active-assisted range-of-motion exercises by helping the client finish the full range of motion. Another form of active-assisted exercise is when a client uses the strong arm to exercise the weaker or paralyzed arm.

ROM exercises remain the same regardless of the degree of assistance required by the client. Active ROM exercises should be encouraged if the client's health status allows because this involves the client in self-care and increases independence and self-esteem. Active and active-assisted ROM exercises help prevent muscular atrophy and joint contracture. Passive ROM exercises help maintain joint function but do not exert enough muscle tension to maintain muscle tone.

Range-of-motion exercises are shown in Table 14. When caring for a client with decreased mobility, keep in mind the following considerations (Perry & Potter, 1994):

1. Assess the family or primary caregiver's ability, availability, and motivation to assist client with exercises client is unable to perform independently.
2. Assist the family or primary caregiver to arrange home environment to promote exercise program, for example, space allocation, lighting, and temperature.
3. Instruct client or caregiver in performing exercises slowly.
4. Teach caregiver how to provide adequate support to joint being exercised.
5. Instruct client to exercise only to point of resistance and to stop if client expresses pain.
6. Provide opportunity for return demonstration.
7. Consult with a physical therapist for additional assistance or exercises and client's response to exercise program.
8. Develop a schedule for recording the performance of the exercise program.
9. An older adult may need ROM exercising broken into two or more sessions to control fatigue.
10. Active ROM exercises can be incorporated into activities of daily living (Table 15), as well as into children's play activities.

Table 14 Range-of-Motion Exercises

Body Part	Type of Joint	Type of Movement
Neck and cervical spine	Pivotal	Flexion: bring chin to rest on chest Extension: return head to erect position Hyperextension: bend head back as far as possible
		Lateral flexion: tilt head as far as possible toward each shoulder
		Rotation: turn head as far as possible to right and left
Shoulder	Ball and socket	Flexion: raise arm from side position forward to position above head Extension: return arm to position at side of the body Hyperextension: move arm behind body, keeping elbow straight
		Abduction: raise arm to side to position above head with palm away from head Adduction: lower arm sideways and across body as far as possible

(Continued)

Table 14   Range-of-Motion Exercises (cont'd)

Body Part	Type of Joint	Type of Movement
		Internal rotation: with elbow flexed, rotate shoulder by moving arm until thumb is turned inward and toward back
		External rotation: with elbow fixed, move arm until thumb is upward and lateral to head
		Circumduction: move arm in full circle. Circumduction is combination of all movements of ball-and-socket joint
Elbow	Hinge	Flexion: bend elbow so that lower arm moves toward its shoulder joint and hand is level with shoulder
		Extension: straighten elbow by lowering hand
		Hyperextension: bend lower arm back as far as possible
Forearm	Pivotal	Supination: turn lower arm and hand so that palm is up
		Pronation: turn lower arm so that palm is down

(Continued)

Table 14   Range-of-Motion Exercises (cont'd)

Body Part	Type of Joint	Type of Movement
Wrist	Condyloid	Flexion: move palm toward inner aspect of the forearm
		Extension: move fingers so that fingers, hands, and forearm are in same plane
		Hyperextension: bring dorsal surface of hand back as far as possible
		Radial flexion: bend wrist medially toward thumb
		Ulnar flexion: bend wrist laterally toward fifth digit
Fingers	Condyloid hinge	Flexion: make fist
		Extension: straighten fingers
		Hyperextension: bend fingers back as far as possible
		Abduction: spread fingers apart
		Adduction: bring fingers together
Thumb	Saddle	Flexion: move thumb across palmar surface of hand
		Extension: move thumb straight away from hand
		Abduction: extend thumb laterally (usually done when placing fingers in abduction and adduction)
		Adduction: move thumb back toward hand
		Opposition: touch thumb to each finger of same hand

(Continued)

Table 14   Range-of-Motion Exercises (cont'd)

Body Part	Type of Joint	Type of Movement
Hip	Ball and socket	Flexion: move leg forward and up Extension: move leg back beside other leg
		Hyperextension: move leg behind body
		Abduction: move leg laterally away from body Adduction: move leg back toward medial position and beyond if possible
		Internal rotation: turn foot and leg toward other leg External rotation: turn foot and leg away from other leg

(Continued)

Table 14   Range-of-Motion Exercises (cont'd)

Body Part	Type of Joint	Type of Movement
		Circumduction: move leg in circle
Knee	Hinge	Flexion: bring heel back toward back of thigh Extension: return heel to floor
Ankle	Hinge	Dorsal flexion: move foot so that toes are pointed upward Plantar flexion: move foot so that toes are pointed downward
Foot	Gliding	Inversion: turn sole of foot medially Eversion: turn sole of foot laterally

(Continued)

Table 14   Range-of-Motion Exercises (cont'd)

Body Part	Type of Joint	Type of Movement
Toes	Condyloid	Flexion: curl toes downward Extension: straighten toes
		Abduction: spread toes apart Adduction: bring toes together

Perry AG and Potter PA: *Clinical nursing skills and techniques, ed. 3*, St. Louis, 1994, Mosby-Year Book, Inc.

Table 15   Incorporating Active Range-of-Joint-Motion Exercises into Activities of Daily Living

Joint Exercised	Activity of Daily Living	Movement
Neck	Nodding head yes	Flexion
	Shaking head no	Rotation
	Moving right ear to right shoulder	Lateral flexion
	Moving left ear to left shoulder	Lateral flexion
Shoulder	Reaching to turn on overhead light	Extension
	Reaching to bedside stand for book	Extension
	Scratching back	Hyperextension
	Rotating shoulders toward chest	Abduction
	Rotating shoulders toward back	Adduction
Elbow	Eating, bathing, shaving, grooming	Flexion, extension
Wrist	Eating, bathing, shaving, grooming	Flexion, extension, hyperextension, abduction, adduction
Fingers/ Thumb	All activities requiring fine motor coordination, e.g., writing, eating, hobbies	Flexion, extension, abduction, adduction, opposition

(Continued)

Table 15   Incorporating Active Range-of-Joint-Motion Exercises into Activities of Daily Living (cont'd)

Joint Exercised	Activity of Daily Living	Movement
Hip	Walking	Flexion, extension, hyperextension
	Moving to side-lying position	Flexion, extension, abduction
	Moving from side-lying position	Extension, adduction
	Rolling feet inward	Internal rotation
	Rolling feet outward	External rotation
Knee	Walking	Flexion, extension
	Moving to and from a side-lying position	Flexion, extension
Ankle	Walking	Dorsiflexion, plantar flexion
	Moving toe toward head of bed	Dorsiflexion
	Moving toe toward foot of bed	Plantar flexion
Toes	Walking	Extension, hyperextension
	Wiggling toes	Abduction, adduction

Perry AG and Potter PA: *Clinical nursing skills and techniques, ed. 3*, St. Louis, 1994, Mosby-Year Book, Inc.

Medication Administration

Medications commonly administered in the home include those given orally, sublingually, topically, intramuscularly, subcutaneously, intravenously, and by inhalation — and that are prescribed by a physician to treat one or more conditions. These drugs are usually scheduled for regular administration or in response to a client request when needed. One of the major nursing responsibilities for medication administration in the home is teaching the client to self-administer the medication to ensure safe, effective results from the therapy. This includes instruction in dosage, route, frequency, time, form, side effects to report, methods of administration, and safe storage.

Assessment

- Age, weight
- Medications taken, both prescribed and OTC
- Drug allergies
- Compatibility of medications being taken; compatibility with foods
- Past dependency or risk for present dependency on drugs
- Use of alcohol, caffeine-containing beverages, herbal products, and tobacco
- Daily routines and best times for medication administration
- Information about each drug and special recommendations for administration
- Ability to swallow tablets
- Cognitive and mental capacities
- Expiration dates of medication, where medications are kept and if kept separate from other drugs in home

Interventions

- Prepare medications in labeled containers; assemble water, food, or anything else needed for administration (e.g., pill crusher if needed and if medication does not need to be swallowed whole).
- Check medications for correct name, dosage, route, and time. Formulate a checklist for client to use that includes time schedules that revolve around daily routines.

- Check drug dosage before, during, and after administration to ensure accuracy; compare with checklist or drug container.
- Prepare drug(s) by pouring liquids, placing tablet in cup or in hand or crushing and mixing with water or in food such as applesauce, or uncapping ointment and squeezing small amount to discard.
- Offer medication to client, using the appropriate aid, e.g., with a glass of water or other fluid to swallow, mixed in food to swallow, or in a measured cup for drinking; or direct patient to apply to affected area with applicator or to place medication under tongue or in the cheek.
- Document administration of medication(s) on checklist.
- Note any side effects and instruct client to report any to the physician.
- Store medications in safe area away from children.
- Follow special instructions in administering a medication, such as taking before or after a meal or using a straw.
- For metered dose inhalant administration, follow special instructions included in the insert.
- Suggest and instruct client in how to use reminder devices (with compartments for drugs that match administration times) and how to refill daily.
- Inform client that if drug is forgotten, wait until next dosage time unless dose can be taken within 1 hour after scheduled time (this will depend on frequency of dosage).

Evaluation

- Client uses checklist and administers drug(s) accurately.
- Client uses reminder devices effectively and refills them daily.
- Client knows drug action, dosage, frequency, route, form, side effects, and incompatibilities with foods and other drugs.
- Client takes preventive measures and stores drugs safely.
- Client reports side effects to physician and stops medication until physician is notified.

Table 16   Assisting Clients in Taking Medications at Home

The following categories are areas in which clients may need support in taking medications at home. Strategies are to be used by the nurse.

Problem Category	Strategy
Understanding schedule and route	Provide adequate oral explanation. Give simple written instructions.
	Suggest using a daily tear-off calendar for once-a-day medication, tearing off page when medication is taken.
	Use larger calendar for multiple medications, placing a checkmark in the dated square after taking each medication.
	Put each medication in a transparent envelope and attach to dated squares. Write name of medicine, time, and dose to be taken on that day.
	Obtain a commercial drug caddy for client with multiple medication needs for a day or week (or use an egg carton).
	Seek or write simple pamphlets and booklets in appropriate language, e.g., English or Spanish. Take into account age, sight, and memory changes of ill clients.
	Use simple audio-visual aids for teaching about medications, medication effects, and proper medication taking.
Opening the bottle	Request pharmacists to place medications in screw- or flip-top container rather than "childproof" container.

(Continued)

Table 16   Assisting Clients in Taking Medications at Home (cont'd)

Problem Category	Strategy
Reading the label	Ask pharmacist to place medications in oversized bottle and prepare label with large print.
	Ask pharmacist to write directions in simple terms and appropriate language, e.g., English, Spanish, etc.
	Devise a color code for multiple medications and include the color key to be kept with medications.
	For visually impaired, seek Braille labels for clients.
Taking too much or too little	Adjust medication schedule to life pattern and habits of client.
	Ask physician to give medication dosages which can be taken at morning and bedtime (2x daily).
	Ask physician to give multiple medications, all of which can be taken at the same times each day.
	Check with physician and pharmacist about compatibility of these multiple drugs and potential drug interactions.
	Monitor effects of medication and ask physician to discontinue medicine as soon as possible if client not compliant.
Difficulty swallowing medications	Ask if medication comes in liquid form and change from tablet/capsules.
	Teach client to put tablet on *back* of tongue and take with fluid.
	Teach client to put capsule on *front* of tongue and take with liquid.

(Continued)

Table 16   Assisting Clients in Taking Medications at Home (cont'd)

Problem Category	Strategy
	Teach client to avoid crushing coated, beaded, plastic matrix tablets and layered tablets.

Modified from Ebersole P and Hess P: *Toward healthy aging, ed. 3*, St. Louis, 1990, Mosby-Year Book, Inc.

Intravenous Medications

Intravenous therapy is initiated for the following reasons (Rice, 1992):

- To replace fluids and correct electrolyte imbalances in dehydrated clients
- To replace fluids and electrolytes lost as a result of vomiting, diarrhea, suctioning, wound drainage, or blood loss
- To provide caloric value for the malnourished or for those who cannot eat
- To administer IV medications such as antibiotics, chemotherapy, or blood products

Client/caregiver education is an essential component of successful home infusion therapy. The client and/or caregiver must be able to demonstrate administration techniques, express a willingness to comply with techniques, understand the signs and symptoms of therapy complications, and be able to identify appropriate interventions. The goal is to enable clients or caregivers to manage long-term home infusion safely with minimal intervention by home health nurses.

Clients and caregivers are taught how to initiate or discontinue the IV therapy, how to flush the catheter, and how to prepare IV fluids for administration. In addition, clients and caregivers are generally taught maintenance and operation of infusion pumps. This includes changing the battery, starting and stopping the pump, and responding appropriately to alarm signals. Finally, clients and caregivers must be taught how to deal with complications of IV therapy. Table 17 provides patient education guidelines for troubleshooting IV therapy in the home.

Table 17   Troubleshooting IV Therapy in the Home: Client/Family Education

Complication	Action
Infusion slows or stops	Observe for swelling, pain, or hardness around needle/catheter site. If any of these are noted, stop the infusion and immediately notify the home health nurse and/or physician. If the above signs and symptoms are not present: 1. Check for twisted tubing or pressure on tubing. 2. See if the client has moved or bent his or her arm. If so, return arm to original position. 3. If the flow rate remains slow or stopped, turn regulator off and contact the home health nurse.
Circulatory overload Occurs when client has received too much fluid. Symptoms: Coughing, shortness of breath Increased respirations	Stop the infusion and immediately call the home health nurse and/or physician. Call an ambulance directly if the situation is an emergency.

(Continued)

Table 17   Troubleshooting IV Therapy in the Home: Client/Family Education (cont'd)

Complication	Action
Headache, facial flushing Rapid pulse rate Dizziness	
Air embolism Air gets into the blood stream. Symptoms: Extreme shortness of breath Anxiety Lips and nailbeds turn blue Rapid pulse rate Loss of consciousness	This is a medical *emergency.* Turn client on left side with head down. Immediately call an ambulance. Stay with the client.
Pyrogenic reaction May occur with exposure to contaminated equipment or solutions	Discontinue IV therapy. Call home health nurse/notify physician.

(Continued)

Table 17   Troubleshooting IV Therapy in the Home: Client/Family Education (cont'd)

Complication	Action
Symptoms: Abrupt temperature, chills Complaints of backache, headache Nausea and vomiting Flushed face Dizziness	Stay with the client until arrival of the home health nurse. (If symptoms are severe, take the client to an emergency department.) Save the equipment/IV solution for laboratory analysis.
Severed catheter	Clamp the line and notify the home health nurse/physician.

From Rice R: *Home health nursing practice: Concepts and application*, St. Louis, 1992, Mosby-Year Book, Inc.

Infection Control

Infection occurs as a result of transmission of an infectious agent to a susceptible host. Home health nurses must keep in mind that an infected individual will not necessarily show signs or symptoms of the infection but may nonetheless be capable of infecting others. Below are common signs and symptoms of infection (Rice, 1992).

Signs and Symptoms of Infection

Inflammatory Response
- Redness
- Heat
- Swelling
- Pain

Other Possible Signs and Symptoms
- Sore throat, cough
- Sputum production, change in color or amount of sputum
- Elevated temperature
- Tachycardia, tachypnea
- Rash, dermatitis of the skin
- Loose stool, diarrhea
- Nausea, vomiting
- Weight loss (inappropriate)
- Green or yellow exudates or drainage from the wound bed
- Burning or painful urination

Understanding mechanisms of transmission provides insight into the management of communicable diseases. The following procedures will reduce the transmission of communicable disease:

- The infectious agent is eradicated by a method of disinfection/sterilization.
- The infectious agent is prevented from entering the host (actual or potential).
- Prevalence of the infectious agent is reduced by enhancing host response by means of antibiotic administration or immunizations.
- The infectious agent's reservoir is neutralized.

These procedures, along with a philosophy that all clients should be treated as though they have an infectious disease, form the basis for infection control guidelines recommended by the Centers for Disease Control (CDC) (Rice, 1992).

Universal Precautions

Universal precautions are those actions taken to prevent transmission of microorganisms from one person to another. They include care of hands, care of inanimate objects or articles used, and use of barriers and techniques to protect against transmission to client or caretaker (Jaffe & Skidmore-Roth, 1993).

Since a health history and physical assessment cannot reliably identify all clients who have a communicable disease, the CDC and OSHA recommend that universal blood and body fluid precautions be followed with all clients. All health care workers should wear gloves when touching mucous membrane or nonintact skin of all clients (e.g., wound care, suctioning care). Masks, goggles, and gowns should be worn if aerosolization or splashes are likely to occur (Rice, 1992).

Provision of Care

- Routine precautions should be taken when there is any possibility of exposure to blood or body fluids of any client (wound care, suctioning, any care involving body orifices or injections). Aprons or gowns are required for procedures involving extensive contact with blood or body fluids. Gloves are required when handling items soiled with blood or body fluids (soiled linens, dressings, catheter/enema equipment).
- Immediately after contact with blood or body fluids all contaminated skin surfaces should be washed completely. Hands should be washed with soap and water immediately after gloves are removed. Wearing gloves does not eliminate the necessity for handwashing after each client contact. Do not reuse disposable gloves. Gloves should be changed between contact with clients to prevent cross-contamination. General utility gloves should not be worn if they are peeling, cracked, or discolored, as this is evidence of deterioration.
- All health care workers who perform or assist in invasive procedures must use extraordinary care to prevent injuries caused by needles, glucose monitoring lancets, and other sharp instruments or devices. After use, disposable syringes, needles, and other sharp items should be placed in a puncture-resistant container for disposal. To prevent needlestick

injuries, needles should not be recapped, purposely bent or broken, removed from disposable syringes, or otherwise bent by hand.

- Although saliva has not been implicated in HIV transmission, mouthpieces or other ventilation devices should be available for employees to minimize the risk involved in emergency mouth-to-mouth resuscitation.
- Health care workers who have exudative lesions, weeping dermatitis, or breaks in the skin should wear gloves when doing any procedural treatment for the client or family.

Disinfection (at the Home Health Agency)

- Wash all equipment thoroughly with soap and water, rinse, and dry.
- Always read the label of the disinfectant and follow directions. After washing equipment with soap and water, disinfect, rinse, and dry. According to OSHA, after initial cleanup one of the following disinfectants should be used for cleaning equipment exposed to blood and/or body substances:
  - Chemical germicides that are approved for use as hospital disinfectants and are tuberculocidal when used at recommended dilutions
  - Products registered by the Environmental Protection Agency (EPA) as being effective against HIV with an accepted "HIV (AIDS Virus)" label
  - A solution of 5.25% sodium hypochlorite (household bleach) diluted between 1:10 and 1:100 with water; mix a fresh supply of bleach every day for effective disinfection
- *Remember:* Disinfectants are designed for inanimate objects and are damaging to the skin. Wear gloves to protect the hands and goggles if there is a possibility of splashes to the eye. Disinfectants should be used in a well-ventilated room. If possible, totally submerge contaminated articles in the disinfecting solution for the required period of time.
- Since most durable medical equipment (DME) used in the home cannot be autoclaved, disinfection is recommended. Submerge or wipe down DME with soap and water and disinfect. Remember, bleach is caustic to metal.

Disposal Techniques for Waste: Environmental Considerations

- Sharps: Injection needles with syringes, glucometer lancets, vacutainer needles, etc., should be contained in a puncture-resistant container marked with the biohazard symbol and sealed to prevent leakage.
- Blood, body fluids, and secretions generated by clients in their own homes may be disposed of via the sanitary sewer.
- All antineoplastic chemotherapeutic wastes are considered a hazardous waste by most health departments and must be neutralized by dilution. Review regulations with local health departments and the EPA.

Special Precautions in Home Care

These guidelines are based on practical adaptations of universal/body substance isolation (BSI) precautions for home health nurses and may be individualized to meet specific client needs.

Provision of Care for Clients with Communicable Diseases

- Explain all procedures and their rationale to clients. Respect clients' rights to privacy and confidentiality.
- Wash hands with soap and water before and after client care and during care if soiled.
- Wear gloves on both hands whenever there is any possibility of contact with blood or body substances (oral or body secretions, feces, urine, vomitus, tissues, wound or other drainage). Change gloves between procedures as appropriate.
- Wear a mask if clients are coughing productively or when suctioning. Masks may be worn if the client has active TB, influenza, mumps, measles, chicken pox, or pertussis.
- Routinely wipe down the bell/diaphragm of the stethoscope with an alcohol prep-pad between clients.
- Do not recap used syringes/needles; place them in a puncture-resistant container for storage.
- Wipe down blood specimen tubes with a 10% bleach solution, if possible; otherwise, use an alcohol prep-pad. Label tube "blood precautions" and store in a sealed plastic bag for laboratory delivery.
- Do not replace any contaminated equipment in the nursing bag until it has been disinfected.

Table 18 Guidelines for Handwashing and Protective Wear

Procedure	Wash Hands	Gloves	Gown	Mask	Eyewear
Talking with clients					
Adjusting IV fluid rate or noninvasive equipment					
Examining client without touching blood, body fluids, or mucous membranes	X				
Examining client with significant cough	X			X	
Examining client including contact with blood, body fluids, mucous membranes, or drainage	X	X			
Drawing blood	X	X			
Inserting venous access	X	X			
Suctioning	X	X	Use gown, mask, and eyewear if blood and/or body fluid spattering is likely		
Inserting body or face catheters	X	X	Use gown, mask, and eyewear if blood and/or body fluid spattering is likely		
Handling soiled waste, linen, or other materials	X	X	Use gown, mask, and eyewear only if waste or linen is extensively contaminated and spattering is likely		

(Continued)

Table 18   Guidelines for Handwashing and Protective Wear (cont'd)

Procedure	Wash Hands	Gloves	Gown	Mask	Eyewear
Intubation	X	X	X	X	X
Inserting arterial access	X	X	X	X	X
Endoscopy, bronchoscopy	X	X	X	X	X
Operative and other procedures that produce extensive spattering of blood and/or body fluids and are likely to soil clothes	X	X	X	X	X

Seidel HM, Ball JB, Dains JE, and Benedict GW: *Mosby's guide to physical examination, ed. 2*, St. Louis, 1991, Mosby–Year Book, Inc.

■ Disinfection methods in the home setting vary. All items to be disinfected should be cleaned first with a detergent and running water. The following are cited as disinfectants used in home care: bleach, white vinegar, hydrogen peroxide, boiling water, phenolics, and isopropyl alcohol. The item to be disinfected will primarily determine the disinfectant to be used. Bleach corrodes metal but is cited as an all-purpose disinfectant in the home for blood and body fluid contamination. White vinegar (acetic acid) may be used to disinfect respiratory therapy equipment, although DME vendor guidelines for cleaning respiratory therapy equipment should be reviewed.

■ Contaminated equipment that cannot be cleaned in the home should be placed in a plastic bag and transported to the agency for disinfection or left in the client's home for exclusive use with that client. (Disposable equipment should be used whenever possible.)

■ Place disposable contaminated items (dressings, etc.) in a plastic bag, seal the bag, and place it in the trash.

■ Pour contaminated liquids (urine, stool, vomitus) into a toilet, followed immediately with full-strength bleach and flushing.

■ Visit clients with communicable diseases last or at the end of the work day.

■ Take only needed equipment/supplies into the home.

■ Documentation should include:
  ■ Client's overall status and vital signs
  ■ Infection control precautions utilized
  ■ Any teaching done with client/caregiver regarding understanding of infection and mechanism of transmission as well as participation and compliance with infection control recommendations

Specific Home Health Agency Precautions Regarding Infection Control

In addition to general recommendations for infection control procedures during the client visit, the following specific recommendations are suggested:

Equipment

■ If using a baby scale, wipe the scale down with disinfectant between uses or use a fresh disposable plastic sheath/pad underneath the baby on each visit.

- For glucose monitors, follow specific manufacturer's guidelines for cleaning.
- If clients do not have their own thermometer, wipe the thermometer with an alcohol prep-pad before and after use and place a plastic/protective sheath over the thermometer before administration to a client.

Bag Technique and Initial Handwashing

Proper technique should be observed at all times:
- The inside of the nursing bag should be regarded as a clean area.
- The bag should be transported in the car on top of a supply of newspapers.
- Once in the client's home, select the cleanest or most convenient area and spread newspaper.
- Place the bag on the newspaper.
- Prepare a receptacle (trash bag) for disposable items.
- Open the nursing bag, and remove items needed to wash hands. Handwashing supplies should be placed at the top of the bag.
- Close the bag. Go in and out of the nursing bag as few times as possible.
- Take items to wash hands (liquid soap/paper towels) to the sink area and wash hands (see separate section on handwashing procedure).
- Return to the bag, open it again, and remove necessary items for the visit.
- Keep the bag closed during the visit. Leave all plastic containers in the bag. Do not reenter the bag unless your hands are clean.
- If a plastic apron is worn, do not return it to the nursing bag. Remove the apron by folding the exposed side inward and discard it along with newspaper and other used, disposable items in the client's waste receptacle.
- The nursing bag should not be exposed to extreme temperatures or left in the car for long periods of time. Nursing bags should be cleaned, disinfected, and restocked weekly at the home health agency.

Disposal of Soiled Dressings

- Place contaminated dressings and disposable supplies in a plastic bag for disposal. Disinfection with a 10% bleach solution before disposal is recommended.
- Seal the plastic bag and place it in the trash.

- The client is responsible for waste disposal in the home setting.
- The nurse is responsible for educating the client regarding neutralization of infectious waste and safe disposal procedures.
- Review local ordinances regarding infectious waste disposal in the home.

Handwashing

To prevent cross-contamination between clients and staff, wash hands *before* and *after* care of client. Handwashing is more thoroughly covered on page 163. However, these basic steps and related precautions should be observed:

- If wearing gloves, *wash hands after removal of gloves.* When providing routine client care, wash hands vigorously under a stream of water for at least 10 seconds.
- If providing care for a client on specific isolation orders, consider use of Betadine scrub.
- Avoid using cloth towels or bars of soap, as these may become a haven for bacteria.
- If running water or clean facilities are not available, hands should be cleaned with an antiseptic foam or rinse.
- Remember, good handwashing technique prevents client cross-contamination.

Contaminated Wound Precautions

- Wash hands. Wear a disposable apron to protect clothing from contamination by drainage or body secretions. Use disposable gloves on both hands. With aseptic technique, follow wound care protocol per physician orders. When procedure is completed, remove apron and gloves and discard into a plastic bag, secure the top, and seal. Wash hands.

Needlestick

Persons who handle needles are at high risk for needlestick injuries. If a needlestick injury occurs:

- Wash the affected area (usually the hands) thoroughly with soap and water. Dry.
- Report the incident to your manager for follow-up and evaluation. An incident report form should be completed.

Sharps Containers

Contaminated needles are to be placed in a puncture-resistant container in the home.

- Clients receiving frequent intravenous therapy should have their own sharps container in their home. (This is often issued and removed for disposal by the intravenous equipment supplier.)
- Sharps containers may be charged to individual clients who require frequent drawing of blood or injections. In addition, home health nurses should have a sharps container issued to them for multiple client use.
- Sharps containers should not be filled to where needles protrude out the opening, as this increases risk of injury.
- When full, return the container to a special hazardous waste receptacle at the home health agency and requisition a new sharps container.

Client Education

As stated previously, client education is a major focus of home health nurses when providing care. Home health nurses should instruct the client and caregiver about infectious disease, mechanisms of transmission, and specific infection control procedures such as proper techniques in handwashing and needle disposal.

Although home health nurses should use sterile technique when performing all procedural care, clean technique can be taught to the client and caregiver when managing illness at home. Information must be imparted so that the client and caregiver can safely manage infectious disease in the home. The home itself becomes another variable in client management. With this in mind, the following guidelines are recommended:

Bathroom

- When others must share a bathroom with a client whose disease is spread by stool, request that the client cover the faucet and handles with tissue paper before touching them.
- The client should also use a separate toothbrush and drinking glass.
- The person cleaning the bathroom should wear rubber gloves; the gloves should be disinfected with a 10% bleach solution after use; and cracked or torn rubber gloves should be discarded.
- Damp towels and wash cloths should be removed as quickly as possible.
- Recommend that the family use a liquid soap. If the client has an outdoor toilet, 3 to 4 cups of lime should be placed in the toilet weekly.

Kitchen

- Instruct the family to keep the refrigerator clean and set the temperature at 45° F.
- Weekly cleaning of the inside of the refrigerator with regular household cleaning agents will help control microbial growth.
- There is no need to prepare the client's food with separate cooking utensils, but clients should be discouraged from sharing the food off their plate with other members of the household.
- The client's utensils and dishes do not necessarily need to be isolated from those used by other household members if they are washed thoroughly with hot, soapy water. However, the use of common or unclean eating utensils should be avoided. Instruct household members to wash the client's dishes last and then disinfect the sink with a 10% bleach solution.

Laundry

- Soiled linen should be handled as little as possible and should be bagged at the location where it was used.
- Caregivers should be instructed to store infected linen in a separate, leakproof plastic bag and to keep the bag tied shut.
- Hands should be washed immediately after handling soiled laundry to prevent spread of infection.
- Contaminated linens should be washed separately from household laundry in extremely hot water (160° F for 25 minutes). One cup of household bleach in addition to the detergent should be added to each load of laundry. The wash cycle should be run through twice, and then the laundry should be dried.
- To clean the washer, the caregiver should run the empty machine through a complete cycle using a commercial disinfectant or 1 cup of full-strength bleach.
- Rubber gloves should be worn when handwashing soiled laundry and then disinfected with a 10% bleach solution.

Client's Room

- Encourage daily cleaning of the room.
- Items such as toys, books, and games may be cleaned with soap and water or wiped down with alcohol.
- Trash containers should be washed with soap and water and sprayed with commercial disinfectant.
- Floors and furniture should be washed with germicidal solution.

- The room should be aired out, if possible.

Personal Hygiene

- Clients should be taught to wash their hands in soap and water before and after evacuating bowels or bladder and before handling food. They should cover their mouth when coughing or sneezing and then wash their hands.
- Paper or tissues used by a client experiencing a productive cough need to be discarded into a plastic garbage bag.
- Caregivers should wash their hands before and after delivery of client care.
- The client's body should be kept clean with soap and water baths.
- Gloves should be worn whenever there is a possibility of touching a client's blood or body substances.

Pets

- Pets sometimes harbor organisms (in excreta or hair) that may pose a threat of serious illness to someone with a compromised immune system.
- AIDS clients in particular should not be responsible for cleaning the bird cage, cat litter box, or fish tank.

Other

- Soiled bedpans and commodes should be cleaned with bleach or household detergent and hot water.
- Disposable supplies used during client care should be placed in a separate plastic bag from the rest of the family trash and sealed.
- Sharps containers should be stored in an area that is inaccessible to children or to others who may be injured by them.
- Both plastic bags and needle containers should be disposed of in compliance with local public health department and community waste disposal regulations. Usually, the regular trash disposal system can be used, but local authorities should be consulted if there are any questions.

Handwashing Technique[*]

1. Use a sink with warm running water, soap, and paper towels.
2. Push wristwatch and long sleeves up above wrist. Remove jewelry, except a plain band, from fingers and arms.
3. Keep fingernails short and filed.
4. Inspect the surface of the hands and fingers for breaks or cuts in the skin and cuticles. Report such lesions when caring for highly susceptible clients.
5. Stand in front of the sink, keeping hands and clothing away from the sink surface. (If hands touch the sink during handwashing, repeat the process.) Use a sink where it is comfortable to reach the faucet.
6. Turn on the water. Turn on hand-operated faucets by covering the faucet with a paper towel.
7. Avoid splashing water against your uniform or clothes.
8. Regulate flow of water so that the temperature is warm.
9. Wet hands and lower arms thoroughly under running water. Keep the hands and forearms lower than the elbows during washing.
10. Apply 1 ml of regular or 3 ml of antiseptic liquid soap to the hands, lathering thoroughly. If bar soap is used, hold it throughout the lathering period. Soap granules and leaflet preparations may be used.
11. Wash the hands, using plenty of lather and friction for at least 10 to 15 seconds. Interlace the fingers and rub the palms and back of hands with a circular motion at least 5 times each.
12. If areas underlying fingernails are soiled, clean them with fingernails of the other hand and additional soap or a clean orangewood stick. Do not tear or cut the skin under or around the nail.
13. Rinse hands and wrists thoroughly, keeping hands down and elbows up.
14. Repeat steps 10 through 12 but extend the actual period of washing for 1-, 2-, and 3-minute handwashings.
15. Dry the hands thoroughly from the fingers up to the wrists and forearms.
16. Discard paper towel in proper receptacle.
17. To turn off a hand faucet, use a clean, dry paper towel.

*Modified from Potter PA and Perry AG: *Fundamentals of nursing: Concepts, process, and practice, ed. 3*, St. Louis, 1993, Mosby-Year Book, Inc.

Intermittent Catheterization*

Intermittent bladder catheterization is a method of draining the urinary bladder by inserting a catheter. Emptying the bladder on an intermittent basis permits a more normal functioning of the bladder, and complete emptying of the bladder eliminates the need for an indwelling catheter and prevents urinary incontinence. The procedure in the home setting is done as a clean technique. Sometimes it is taught to the client before discharge from the hospital or long-term care facility.

Short-Term Goals

The client will:
- Be able to perform self-catheterization using clean technique.
- Have basic knowledge of fluid balance and signs and symptoms of infection.
- Understand the importance of personal hygiene, such as handwashing.

Long-Term Goals

- The client will be able to incorporate intermittent catheterization into the lifestyle with minimal interruption.
- The client will demonstrate compliance in all aspects of management of bladder emptying to prevent recurrent infection and encourage possible return of function of the bladder.

Nursing Assessment

- The client must be assessed for ability to manage the procedure and understand all aspects of care.
- The pattern for self-catheterization should be determined, taking into consideration the client's planned lifestyle. The client may need to do the procedure every 4 hours and thus must be near a bathroom suitable for the procedure.

*Beare PG and Myers JL: *Principles and practice of adult health nursing,* ed. 2, St. Louis, 1994, Mosby-Year Book, Inc.

Client education should include the following:

- Equipment needed includes a catheter and water-soluble lubricant, soap and warm water, and cloths for carrying the catheter.
- A urinal or other large container with measurements marked in ounces to measure the amount of urine is recommended for clients who are doing self-catheterization for residual urine.
- Handwashing for 5 minutes with soap and warm water must be done before handling the clean catheter.
- The catheter can be reused several times; thus it must be washed with soap and warm water, drained, and allowed to dry. The catheter can be carried in a clean cloth such as a washcloth.
- The need for increased fluid intake must be stressed to ensure fluid balance.
- Scheduling of the procedure and the need for regular self-catheterization should also be stressed, because the client will not feel bladder distention or the need to void.
- The signs and symptoms of urinary tract infection are included in teaching. Signs such as cloudy urine or foul-smelling urine or fever may indicate bladder problems. Changes in bowel patterns, such as diarrhea, may also indicate a bladder problem and thus should not be ignored. Bladder discomfort or pain will not be felt by the client; therefore, the other signs and symptoms are important.

The following information should be used as a guide for client teaching:

- Female catheterization: For a woman with poor vision this may be a very difficult procedure to perform. The procedure can be done while sitting on the toilet or commode or by placing the open end of the catheter into a urinal. The client should wash her hands before beginning the procedure. She should then take the following steps:
  1. Lubricate the tip of the catheter.
  2. Wash the perineal area with soap and water.
  3. Wash hands well with warm soapy water, rinse, and dry.
  4. Take the catheter in one hand 2 to 3 inches from the tip.
  5. Spread the labia apart and insert the catheter into the meatus. This procedure will take practice, and a mirror may help the client locate the meatus.
  6. Insert the catheter until a flow of urine starts.

7. When the stream of urine slows, press the lower abdomen to completely empty the bladder.

8. Remove the catheter slowly.

9. If necessary, measure the collected urine, and record the amount.

10. Make other observations such as blood in the urine, foul odor, or increased cloudiness of the urine. Notify the physician of any of these observations.

11. Clean the catheter, and store it for the next use.

■ Male catheterization: This procedure can be done over a toilet or commode or by draining the urine into a urinal. The client should wash his hands before starting the procedure.

1. Generously lubricate the tip of the catheter.

2. Wash the penis well with soap and water.

3. Wash hands with warm soapy water, rinse, and dry.

4. Pick up the catheter 2 to 3 inches from the tip.

5. Insert the catheter into the meatus, and slowly insert the catheter until a flow of urine starts from the end of the catheter.

6. When the stream slows, gently press on the lower abdomen to empty the bladder.

7. Remove the catheter slowly.

8. If necessary, measure the urine, and record the amount.

9. Make other observations such as blood in the urine, a foul odor, or increased cloudiness. Notify the physician of any of these observations.

10. Clean the catheter, and store it for the next use.

Intravenous Fluid Hydration*

Intravenous fluid and electrolyte replacement is indicated when a patient cannot take fluids by mouth or through tube feedings. This therapy is sometimes used as a palliative care measure along with other terminal care. Other forms of intravenous therapy such as total parenteral nutrition or chemotherapy are discussed elsewhere in this book.

Short-Term Goals

- All necessary equipment will be available.
- The caregiver and/or client will have basic knowledge of the procedures for administering intravenous therapy in the home setting.

Long-Term Goals

- The client will receive adequate hydration to maintain fluid and electrolyte balance.
- The caregiver will be able to incorporate intravenous therapy into the total care plan with the assistance of a home health nurse.

Nursing Assessment

Health Management Pattern

A person must be available as a primary caregiver for the duration of the home therapy.

Cognitive Pattern

The caregiver and/or client must demonstrate sufficient skill to be able to learn and manage intravenous therapy equipment and procedures.

Coping/Stress Tolerance Pattern

The total care plan for the client must be reviewed; since clients needing hydration usually have other care needs, the caregiver may perceive hydration as a "high-tech" procedure and may be-

*Beare PG and Myers JL: *Principles and practice of adult health nursing,* ed. 2, St. Louis, 1994, Mosby-Year Book, Inc.

become overwhelmed and thus unable to manage the basic needs for the client.

Resources

Financial and insurance resources must be investigated before ordering intravenous therapy for the home; the caregiver and client need to supply all available insurance information to the home care agencies to determine the source of payment for therapy at home.

Environmental

Evaluation of the home environment may be needed before IV fluid hydration in the home can begin; there is a need for storage space for supplies and bathroom facilities for handwashing. The location of the home and the accessibility for delivery of supplies and provision of 24-hour on-call nursing services by an intravenous therapy nurse must be assessed.

Planning

Therapeutic plan

The physician must write orders for the amount and type of fluids and electrolytes and the rate of administration; if the client is relatively stable, the rate may be such that the 24-hour total volume can be given over an 8-, 10-, or 12-hour period. The schedule can be adapted to the other needs of the client: for example, the client can be given fluid for 12 hours during the night to allow flexibility during the day or 12 hours during the day to allow for monitoring of the fluid and allow the caregiver to have uninterrupted sleep during the night.

Caregiver Education

Education should be scheduled to allow the caregiver a minimum of two or three teaching sessions; instruction should be done with the equipment that will be used.

Implementation

The following information should be included in the client education:

- Use of the equipment, including the administration set, needles, syringes, catheter plug, solution bags, and intravenous pump

- How to check for sterility of supplies and for particulate matter or cloudiness of the solution
- The procedure for site care, either peripheral or central
- How to start and discontinue the intravenous therapy
- How to calculate and monitor the fluid rate
- How to safely discard equipment after use
- How and when to reorder supplies
- How to monitor for local infection such as phlebitis or cellulitis
- How to monitor intake and output
- The necessity for handwashing and the prevention of contamination of the site, the supplies, and the solution

It is advisable to leave written instructions in the home.

Venous Access Devices

The three most frequently used venous access devices are heparin locks, central venous catheters, and implantable devices. It is essential to know how to use and take care of these devices and the equipment needed for their use.

Heparin Lock

This venous access device consists of a short needle or catheter inserted in a peripheral vein, usually in the hand or arm. It is secured to the skin by tape or a transparent dressing (Figure 2).

Site care consists of observing the site, cleansing it with an antiseptic solution, and reapplying a clean transparent dressing. The frequency of dressing changes depends on the type of dressing used, the condition of the patient's skin, and the patient's general health status.

The frequency of flushing the device depends on the frequency of medications and/or fluids, the physician's preference, and the recommendations of the device's manufacturer. The short catheter is flushed after the drug is administered. Because it is in a peripheral site, there is minimal danger of clotting; therefore, frequent flushing with heparin is not necessary. Frequent gentle flushing (at least once every 24 hours at home) may be necessary if the client has poor vein access and if finding another site would be difficult.

Equipment needed includes tape; transparent dressings; sterile catheter plug; heparin flush, saline flush in a syringe with needle (if available), or separate disposable syringes; alcohol wipe to clean catheter plug before flushing; and antiseptic solution for cleansing the site. Because this is a peripheral site in a small vein, arrangements must be made before discharge to have the site changed by a skilled IV therapy nurse on a regular basis and as needed. The site should be checked every few days by a home health nurse or on return to a clinic or physician's office.

Central Venous Catheters

The central venous catheter is a large-bore catheter with one, two, or three ports that can be used for administering medications and/or fluids. The catheter is tunneled under the skin and into the superior vena cava. Medications administered through this catheter are mixed with large quantities of blood, thus decreasing the local reaction to drugs. The Hickman and Broviac catheters are two of the many types of central venous catheters (Figure 3).

Because the catheter is placed into the superior vena cava, the care of this catheter is very important. It is imperative that aseptic technique be used, and at times sterile technique may be used. Vital aspects of care include cleansing the insertion site to prevent infection, flushing with the recommended solution to prevent formation of clots, and keeping the ports capped to prevent introduction of air into the circulatory system.

Equipment needed includes antiseptic solution, such as povidone iodine or alcohol; external dressing such as a transparent dressing; gloves; tape (these supplies are available in kits that can be ordered for use by the patient at home); and heparin flush syringes with needles and saline flush syringes with needles (the quantity needed will depend on the frequency of flushing ordered by the physician and the number of ports).

Implantable Devices

These devices include such brands as Infusaid Implantable Drug Delivery System (Infusaid Inc., Norwood, Mass.), the Medtronic Drug Administration Device (Medtronic Inc., Minneapolis, Minn.), Port-A-Cath (Pharmacia Deltec Inc., St. Paul, Minn.), Infuse-A-Port (Infusaid) or Mediport (Cormed, Mahar, N.Y.). Because these devices are implanted under the skin, the only care needed is a dry sterile dressing until the site is healed and then regular observation of the skin over the device (Figure 4).

Equipment needed includes dry sterile dressings until the wound has healed; special needles may be necessary to fill the device, and alcohol swabs or other antiseptic solution are necessary to prepare the skin over the device for the insertion of the needle into the reservoir of the pump (Beare & Myers, 1994).

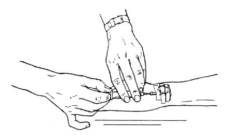

Figure 2 Heparin lock

From Gray DC: Calculate with Confidence, St. Louis, 1994, Mosby-Year Book, Inc.

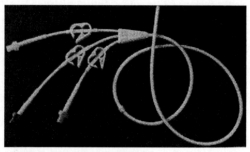

Figure 3 Hickman catheter

Courtesy Davol, Inc., Providence, RI)

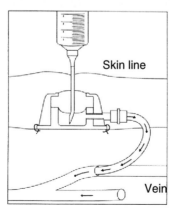

Figure 4 Implanted infusion port

Courtesy Pharmacia Deltec, Inc., St. Paul, MN

Care of
Special Clients

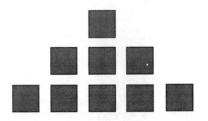

Maternal Care

Over the last several years, hospital stays for childbirth have shortened dramatically. While stays of four to five days were common in the late 1970s, new mothers are now typically discharged 24 to 48 hours after delivery. This has created an increased demand for follow-up visits by a home health agency. For this reason, the home health nurse should be familiar with postpartum assessments and inventory (Bobak, 1993).

Postpartum Assessment

Interview

- Ethnic or cultural variations and nursing actions desired
- Knowledge of hygiene
- Nutrition: amounts taken, food preferences, and knowledge of, for self and family
- Readiness for self-care
  - Extent of skill in self-care
  - Client's need for knowledge of
    1. Breast self-examination
    2. Resumption of sexual intercourse
    3. Contraception
  - Client's need for help at home, acquisition of car seat for newborn, and social assistance (e.g., food stamps)
  - Client's knowledge of
    1. Warning signs and symptoms for which to call the physician
    2. Resources for assistance (e.g., hemorrhage, infection, information such as Tel-Med)

Physical Examination

- Receive report from nurse in labor unit, and review prenatal record if possible.
- Assess physical recovery (Bobak, 1995):
  Breasts
  - Supported by well-fitted brassiere
  - Nontender; no signs of inflammation
  - Intact nipples without cracks, fissures, or undue soreness
  If breastfeeding
  - Describes or demonstrates technique for placing baby on and removing baby from breast, positioning to decrease

stress of nipple area

If not breastfeeding

- No engorgement
- Taking lactation suppressants correctly (if prescribed) and knows warning signs to report
- Discusses importance of not stimulating breasts

Uterus

- Fundus firm, descending below umbilicus approximately 1 cm/day

Bowels/bladder

- Resumption of usual pattern of bowel elimination
- Hemorrhoids (if present) decreasing in size; not causing undue discomfort
- Resumption of usual pattern of urinary elimination; no burning or difficulty in initiating stream

Lochia

- Reveals normally progressing involution—rubra, serosa, alba in decreasing amounts—normal fleshy odor, no clots

Incision: perineal or abdominal

- Episiotomy (if present) well approximated without undue redness, edema, ecchymosis, discharge, or tenderness
- Cesarean incision (if present) clean, dry, well approximated, skin staples, sutures, or Steri-strips intact (if still present); evidence of normal healing process

Legs

- Nontender, with negative Homans' sign bilaterally
- Assess ability to ambulate (both tolerance for and knowledge of need for) and plans for exercise and rest at home.

Laboratory Tests

- Hematocrit (Hct) or packed cell volume (PCV)
- Complete blood count (CBC) if needed
- Urinalysis if needed
- Need for rubella vaccination
- Need for $Rh_o(D)$ immune globulin

Vital Signs

Temperature

- During first 24 hours, may rise to 38° C (100.4° F) as a result of dehydrating effects of labor; after 24 hours the woman should be afebrile
- A diagnosis of puerperal sepsis is suggested if a rise in maternal temperature to 38° C (100.4° F) is noted after the

first 24 hours after birth and recurs or persists for 2 days; other possibilities are mastitis, endometritis, urinary tract infections, and other systemic infections

Pulse

- Bradycardia is a common finding for the first 6 to 8 days after birth; a pulse rate of between 50 and 70 bpm may be considered normal
- Sudden increase: assess for infection, cardiac decompensation, or hemorrhage

Respirations

- Respirations should fall to within the woman's normal pre-birth range
- Decreased rate: may follow an unusually high subarachnoid (spinal) block
- Hyperventilation: assess for anxiety
- Increased rate: assess for cardiac decompensation; may accompany epidural narcotic injection

Blood Pressure

- Blood pressure is altered *slightly*, if at all
- Falling: assess for rising pulse and shock (e.g., hypovolemic shock)
- Rising: assess for signs of preeclampsia/PIH: headache, hyperreflexia; assess amount and type of oxytocic received

Planning and Implementation

- Identify gaps in knowledge and review these points, if necessary:
  - Self-care activities and infant-care activities
  - Warning signs
  - Return of ovulation and menstruation
  - Lactation and weaning or suppression of lactation
  - Resumption of sexual intercourse and fertility management
  - Medications that have been prescribed for the client
- Help the client develop a support system for help with cooking, cleaning, child care, shopping, and so on.
- Identify the need for referral to community resources (e.g., homemaker or child care services, food stamps) and initiate communication with the proper agency or person (social worker), when appropriate.

- Provide the client with a printed instruction sheet that includes phone numbers to call day and night in case of questions or problems.

Postpartum Complications

Temperature ≥ 38° C (100.4° F)

- First 24 hours: assess environment (too hot? too many bedclothes?); offer fluids, or if IV in, leave in TKO; offer food; encourage rest
- After 24 hours: take action as above; assess for signs/symptoms of infection: foul-smelling lochia, URI, UTI, mastitis, or thrombophlebitis; notify physician

Blood Pressure

- Falling: assess for rising pulse and shock (e.g., hypovolemic); report to physician
- Rising: assess for signs of preeclampsia or PIH: headache, hyperreflexia; assess amount and type of oxytocic received; report to physician

Pulse (Heart Rate)

- Bradycardia (50-70 beats/min) (first 6 to 8 days): observe; usually within normal range
- Sudden increase: assess for infection, cardiac decompensation, or hemorrhage

Respirations

- Decreased rate: may follow an unusually high subarachnoid (spinal) block; may accompany epidural narcotic injection: follow protocol (e.g., give naloxone [Narcan])
- Hyperventilation: assess for anxiety
- Increased rate: assess for cardiac decompensation

Uterus

- Deviated from the midline, boggy, remains above the umbilicus after 24 hours

Appetite

- Lack of appetite

Elimination

- Urine: inability to void, urgency, frequency, dysuria
- Bowel: constipation, diarrhea

Rest

- Inability to sleep

Thrombophlebitis (Legs)

- *Superficial:* Vein is swollen, red; palpation over vein reveals a tender cord that feels hard or solid
- *Positive Homans' sign* identifies deeper vein thrombophlebitis; Positive sign: dorsiflexion of foot causes calf muscles to compress tibial veins and produce pain; painful, reddened area; warmth on posterior aspect of calf
- Affected leg may appear larger than unaffected leg
- STAT: Initiate *complete* bed rest with legs elevated
  - Report to physician.
  - Implement physician's orders.

Perineum: Report Immediately

- Perineum: pronounced edema, not intact, marked discomfort
- Lochia: heavy, foul odor
- *Hematoma:* assess for maternal hypovolemic shock
  - Vulvar: swelling in one side; skin purplish over swollen area
  - Vaginal: intense pain; protruding soft mass into vagina or anus
- *Infection:* drainage from sutures; foul odor; increased pulse; chills; increased temperature
- *DIC:* oozing blood or serosanguineous drainage from sutures

Mastitis

- Mass or lump that is painful and hot to touch; increased pulse and temperature; cracked and fissured nipples, inverted nipples
- Record and report to physician

Eclampsia

Assessment

- Measure blood pressure every 4 hours for 48 hours; *even if no convulsions occurred before birth, they may occur within this period.*
- Assess for boggy uterus and a large lochia flow secondary to magnesium sulfate therapy.
- Assess for diuresis (should occur within 72 hours after birth).

- Ask woman to report headaches, blurred vision, etc.; assess affect, alertness, or dullness.

Implementation

- Monitor magnesium sulfate infusion.
- Assess blood pressure before medicating for headache.
- Avoid ergot products (ergonovine maleate)—they increase blood pressure.

Signs of Psychosocial Problems

- Inability or refusal to discuss labor and birth experience
- Refusal to interact with or care for baby (e.g., does not name baby, does not want to hold or feed baby)
- Refusal to attend infant care (including breast-feeding) classes
- Refusal to discuss contraception
- Refers to self as ugly and useless
- Excessive preoccupation with self (body image)
- Marked depression
- Lack of support system

Care of the Neonate

Physiologic Adaption of Infant*

Temperature
- 97.7° to 98.6° F (36.5° to 37° C) axillary route

Heart rate
- 120 to 160 beats/min, strong, regular, normal variations with activity

Respiration
- 30 to 50 breaths/min, normal breath sounds, irregular rhythm; no retractions or grunting; normal variations with activity

Skin
- Warm; good turgor; no rashes

Head
- Symmetric, with flat fontanels; molding or caput decreasing; no hematoma

Abdomen
- Soft, nondistended; audible bowel sounds

Color
- Consistent with racial background; no evidence of jaundice

Activity
- Alert with good muscle tone; moving all extremities normally

Umbilical cord
- Normal atrophy noted; dry base without redness; not malodorous

Circumcision
- Bell in place (if appropriate); clean and healing; no evidence of oozing; urinary stream normal

*From Bobak IM, Jensen MD, and Lowdermilk DL: *Maternity nursing, ed. 4*, St. Louis, 1995, Mosby-Year Book, Inc.

Elimination

- Wetting a minimum of 6 to 10 diapers/day; stools consistent with feeding method in color, number, and consistency

Sleep pattern

- Sleeps well

Feeding

- Sucking well without excessive spitting
- Burping well
- Length of breast-feeding (if done) consistent with recommendations
- Amount of formula per feeding (if done) consistent with recommendations

Table 19   Standard Laboratory Values: Neonatal Period

	Term	Preterm
Hematologic values		
Hemoglobin (g/dL)	17-19	15-17
Hematocrit (%)	57-58	45-55
WBC/mm3	15,000	10,000-20,000

Urinalysis
Volume: 20-40 mL excreted daily in the first few days
Protein: may be present in first 24 days
Casts and WBCs: may be present in first 24 days
Osmolarity (mOsm/L): 100-600
pH: 5-7
Specific gravity: 1.001-1.020

Serum bilirubin
Normal values:
Direct bilirubin: 0.1 to 0.3 mg/dL
Indirect bilirubin: 0.2 to 0.8 mg/dL
Total bilirubin: 0.1 to 1.0 mg/dL
Total bilirubin in newborns: 1 to 12 mg/dL
Phototherapy is usually started if total bilirubin is between 5 and 9 mg/dL in less than 24 hours or between 10 and 14 mg/dL in 24 to 48 hours

Bobak IM and Jensen MD: *Maternity and gynecologic care: The nurse and the family, ed. 5*, St. Louis, 1993, Mosby-Year Book, Inc.

Postoperative Wound Care

Preparing the Patient for Discharge and Home Care

Over the last decade, we have seen increasingly shorter hospital stays even for individuals who have just undergone surgical procedures. Even those receiving abdominal surgery have been known to be either treated in outpatient surgical centers or operated on and released after stays of only one or two days. As a result, more clients than ever are being sent home in need of follow-up care or postoperative wound care in the home. This has created an increasing demand on the home health nurse.

Short-Term Goals

- The client will use, verbalize, and perform basic knowledge of wound care procedures prescribed by the physician.
- All the supplies and equipment needed to carry out procedures will be available.

Long-Term Goals

- The client's wound will heal without complications.
- Wound management will be incorporated into the total care plan of the client.

Nursing Assessment Factors

Health Management Pattern

The client's ability to care for his or her own wound depends on factors such as the location of the wound, which affects the ability to see or reach the wound; the type of wound care involved, such as packing, irrigating, or a simple dry sterile dressing; the client's energy level; and the total care needs of the client. Clients with wounds of the lower extremity may have weight-bearing and ambulation restrictions. Wounds of the upper extremity may make it impossible for the client to perform the wound care since most wound care procedures require two hands.

Cognitive Pattern

The client and/or caregiver must be able to learn the procedure, especially if it is a complex wound management plan.

Therapeutic Plan

The total medical plan must be assessed so that an overall plan can be established. The physician may want a wound to heal by secondary intention; therefore, the packing procedure is very important. The type of antibiotic and the route of administration must be known so that teaching can begin. The physician may plan on an extended course of IV antibiotics and wound care.

Potential for Compliance

Wound healing depends on wound management, taking of all prescribed medications, and completion of all procedures. The client must be aware of the importance of taking medications, especially antibiotics, on a scheduled basis and must be aware of the importance of each of the steps in the irrigation and wound-packing procedure.

Environment

The need for bathroom facilities for handwashing and wound care is very important.

Client Education

Education of the client/caregiver for wound management includes understanding:
- The type of dressings used for all steps in the procedure including the type of dressing for packing a wound, the type for absorbing wound drainage, special dressings that are precut to go around a tube and the type of tape to be used to secure the dressing, and any specific brands of dressings currently used
- Wound irrigation procedures, including the type of irrigation solution used, and the equipment needed to flush the wound and catch the solution as it runs out
- Instructions in sterile technique using gloves and sterilized equipment (included when there is danger of contamination of an open wound)
- Discarding of dressings and irrigation solutions, especially from an infected wound
- How to reorder equipment ahead of time

- Instructions in signs and symptoms of infection, dehiscence, or hemorrhage, along with how and when to seek medical care
- Instructions in wound healing so that the client can recognize steps in the wound healing process

---

Wound Care Guidelines for the Client in the Home Care Setting

After initial treatment and education have begun, the following guidelines may be left with the client:

- Always wash your hands before and after changing your dressing, because good handwashing will help keep your wound clean and prevent the spread of germs.
- Keep all your medical supplies in a clean area; boxes of dressings, gloves, and other medical supplies may be stored in a clean plastic trash bag. Keep all solutions used to clean your wound in the refrigerator after they're opened (this cuts down on the growth of germs). Discard these solutions after 1 week or sooner if you see particles forming in the container or if the solution changes color or becomes cloudy. If you are running out of medical supplies, notify the home health agency.
- Gather up your supplies. Prepare a plastic bag for disposal of dirty dressings and supplies.
- Prepare your new dressing as your home health nurse has instructed you. All caregivers should wear gloves when assisting you with your dressing changes.
- Carefully remove your old dressing and inspect your wound. Any noticeable differences in size, color, or drainage should be reported to the home health nurse or aide at the next visit.
- Apply your new dressing as the home health nurse has shown you. Your dressing should be changed according to schedule or if it comes off or becomes soggy. Place your dirty dressings/supplies in the plastic bag. Seal and dispose of the bag.
- Call the home health agency if you have an elevated temperature or problems with pus or excessive wound drainage or if swelling and pain occur with your wound.

Rice R: *Home health nursing practice: Concepts and application*, St. Louis, 1992, Mosby-Year Book, Inc.

Chemotherapy

Clients requiring chemotherapy may be discharged with various types of venous access devices. These devices allow patients to receive a series of treatments without needing a new IV site for each treatment, thus preserving the veins for future use.

There are two general types of devices: one is surgically implanted under the skin, and the other is a percutaneous device inserted through the skin into a vein. The former requires very little care after the incision has healed and is accessed by a needle inserted through the skin into the device. The percutaneous type, such as a heparin lock or a Hickman catheter, requires specific care on a regular basis. In some cases the venous access device is inserted on an outpatient basis.

Short-Term Goals

- All necessary supplies and equipment will be available.
- The client and caregiver will know basic procedures for caring for the venous access device.

Long-Term Goals

- The client will be able to complete the planned chemotherapy without complications from the venous access device.
- The client will be able to incorporate care of the venous access device into activities of daily living.

Nursing Assessment Factors

- The client's ability to manage care of the venous access site must be assessed. A caregiver may be included for some of the procedures if the client is acutely ill and unable to manage the procedure alone (if the client is elderly, caregiver education is essential).
- Environment—The home environment must to be evaluated. There must be handwashing facilities, accessibility for delivery of supplies and equipment, and provisions for emergency assistance.
- Cognitive pattern—Selecting a venous access device for long-term chemotherapy should be done after assessing the client's ability to care for the device.

- Coping: stress tolerance pattern—The total client care plan must be reviewed. The rate of teaching will be affected by the client's overall ability, the diagnosis, and the total care plan.
- Resources—Financial and insurance resources must be investigated before ordering the necessary equipment. The reimbursement for equipment varies, depending on the skilled care needs of the client, the type of insurance, and where the chemotherapy will be administered.

Client Education

- The length of time needed for teaching depends on the type of access device and the teaching needs of the client.
- Client and caregiver education should allow the client and caregiver a minimum of one or two teaching sessions. The education session should include the following (Beare & Myers, 1994):
  - How to use the equipment, including needles, syringes, heparin flush syringes, and catheter plugs
  - How to check for sterility of supplies
  - The recommended procedure for site care for percutaneous devices
  - How to safely discard equipment after use
  - How and when to reorder equipment
  - How to monitor for local infection, such as phlebitis or cellulitis of either type of device
  - How to distinguish between reaction to the chemotherapeutic agent and a systemic infection
  - The necessity for handwashing and for prevention of contamination of the venous access site
  - The safety precautions regarding capping of the central venous transcutaneous access device
  - A phone number to call if a problem arises

Diabetes Mellitus

Diabetes mellitus is a metabolic disorder affecting a variety of physiologic systems, the most critical of which involves glucose metabolism. The term represents a generalization about a group of anatomic and chemical problems that result from a deficiency of insulin. The most striking abnormality of the disease is the development of fasting hyperglycemia (elevated blood sugar level), hyperlipidemia (elevated blood lipid level), and hyperaminoacidemia (elevated amino acid level). Diabetes mellitus can be caused by an insufficient quantity of secreted insulin or resistance to insulin action.

There are three subclasses of diabetes mellitus. These are (1) insulin-dependent diabetes mellitus (IDDM), or type I (previously called juvenile diabetes); (2) non-insulin-dependent diabetes mellitus (NIDDM), or type II (previously called maturity onset); and (3) other types, such as diabetes secondary to pancreatic disease or drugs or chemical agents. These classifications include diabetes associated with other physical conditions, impaired glucose tolerance, gestational diabetes mellitus, and increased risk of developing diabetes because of previous abnormality of glucose tolerance or potential abnormality of glucose tolerance.

The majority of diabetic patients fall within the IDDM or NIDDM classifications. Table 20 summarizes the classifications and characteristics of diabetes millitus.

Table 20   Classification and Characteristics of Diabetes Mellitus

Name	Previous Synonyms	Characteristics
Type I Insulin-dependent diabetes mellitus (IDDM)	Juvenile diabetes Juvenile onset diabetes Ketosis-prone diabetes Brittle diabetes Idiopathic diabetes	Long preclinical period with abrupt onset of clinical symptoms Individual prone to ketoacidosis Insulin dependent Several syndromes: both primary autoimmune and genetic-environment Often affects young around age of puberty Decrease in size and number of islet cells
Type II Non-insulin-dependent diabetes mellitus (NIDDM)	Adult onset diabetes Maturity onset diabetes Stable diabetes Ketosis-resistant diabetes	Usually not insulin-dependent Individual not ketosis prone (but may form ketones under stress) Multiple syndromes: obese, nonobese, and maturity onset in the young (MODY) Generally occurs in those over age 40 Strong familial pattern being investigated

(Continued)

Table 20   Classification and Characteristics of Diabetes Mellitus (cont'd)

Name	Previous Synonyms	Characteristics
Malnutrition-related diabetes (MRDM)	Tropical diabetes Pancreatic diabetes Pancreatogenic diabetes Endocrine pancreatic syndrome	Seen in tropical, developing countries Seen in young persons with severe protein malnutrition and emaciation Develop severe hyperglycemia without ketosis Uncertain etiology and pathophysiology
Other types	Secondary diabetes	Associated with other conditions/syndromes such as pancreatic disease, hormonal disease, drugs, and chemical agents
Other related conditions		
Impaired glucose tolerance (IGT)	Asymptomatic diabetes Chemical diabetes Borderline diabetes Subclinical diabetes Latent diabetes	Show abnormal response to oral glucose tolerance test; 10% to 15% will convert to type II diabetes within 10 years Many with IGT are obese

(Continued)

Table 20 Classification and Characteristics of Diabetes Mellitus (cont'd)

Name	Previous Synonyms	Characteristics
Gestational diabetes mellitus (GDM)	Same as above	Glucose intolerance first recognized during pregnancy, most likely in the third trimester
		Following pregnancy, glucose may normalize, remain impaired, or progress to diabetes mellitus
		Occurs in 2% of all pregnancies; 60% will develop diabetes mellitus within 15 years of gestation
Statistical risk class		
Previously abnormal glucose level	Latent diabetes Prediabetes	Previous abnormality of oral glucose tolerance or increased risk of developing diabetes because of genetic relationship with a diabetic
Potential abnormal glucose tolerance	Potential diabetes	Family history of diabetes mellitus

McCance KL and Heuther SE: *Pathophysiology: The biological basis for disease in adults and children, ed. 2*, St. Louis, 1994, Mosby-Year Book, Inc.

Diabetic Foot Care

Prevention of ulcers, trauma, and infections of the lower extremities is the key to prevention of amputation. The need for daily foot care, including inspection, cannot be overemphasized. Teach clients to take shoes and stockings off at each medical visit and ask the physician to examine the feet. A podiatric evaluation is recommended for all diabetic clients; podiatric services are essential when there are vascular changes, neuropathy, or foot lesions such as calluses, corns, or bunions.

The following are guidelines for client teaching about proper foot care (Long, 1993):

- Wear well-fitting shoes and clean stockings at all times when walking, and *never walk barefooted*.
- Bathe feet daily and dry them well, paying particular attention to area between the toes.
- Do not self-treat calluses, corns, or ingrown toenails; a podiatrist should be consulted if these are present.
- Bath water should be 29.5° to 32° C (85° to 90° F) and should be tested with a bath thermometer or the elbow before immersing the feet.
- Avoid using heating pads or hot water bottles and warming feet against radiator or close to fireplace.
- Institute measures that help increase circulation to the lower extremities:
  - Avoid smoking.
  - Avoid crossing legs when sitting.
  - Protect extremities when exposed to cold.
  - Avoid immersing feet in cold water.
  - Use socks or stockings that do not apply pressure to the legs at specific sites.
  - Institute a regimen of exercises.
- Inspect feet daily and report any cuts, cracks, redness, blisters, or other signs of trauma to health care provider so that early treatment can be instituted. If necessary, use a mirror to examine the soles.
- If feet are dry, use a lubricating lotion or cream; if moist, use powder.

Table 21   Diabetic Emergencies

Hyperglycemia	Hypoglycemia
Symptoms	
Increased thirst and urination	Shakiness, pounding of heart
Large amounts of sugar and ketones in urine	Excessive sweating, faintness
Blood glucose levels over 300 mg/dL	Headache, impaired vision
Weakness, abdominal pains, generalized aches	Irritability, personality change
Deep breathing	Not able to wake
Loss of appetite, nausea and vomiting	Hunger
Causes	
Too little insulin	Too much insulin
Failure to follow diet	Not eating enough food
Infection, fever	Unusual amount of exercise
Emotional stress	Delayed meal
Treatment	
Give fluid *without* sugar if able to swallow	Take food containing sugar (orange juice, milk, crackers)
Test blood frequently (if possible) for elevated glucose	Do not give fluids if client is not conscious
Test urine frequently for ketones	Get medical assistance immediately if client is not responsive to treatment
Call the doctor	Can give subcutaneous glucagon if available

From Bergenstal R: Acute and chronic complications of diabetes, *Caring* 3(11), November, 1988. Reprinted by permission of the National Association for Home Care.

Respiratory Disorders

Clients with respiratory disorders may suffer from a variety of symptoms, including ineffective airway clearance, ineffective breathing patterns, or impaired gas exchange. These are summarized in Table 22.

Table 22   Etiology, Manifestations, and Treatment of Respiratory Disorders

Disorder/Definition	Cause	Signs	Symptoms	Treatment
OBSTRUCTIVE DISORDERS				
Asthma (*Age group = all ages*)				
Intermittent wheezing, chest tightness, and cough with bronchial hyperresponsiveness *or a* 20% reduction in FEV$_1$ with provocation challenge *or a* 20% increase in FEV$_1$ after inhaled bronchodilator; inflammatory changes in wall of airways	Etiology not clear; interaction between genetic factors (atopy and airway hyperresponsiveness) *or a* environmental factors (allergens, viral infections, pollutants); *extrinsic asthma* usually caused by allergy and starts in childhood; *intrinsic asthma* does not have evidence of allergy and usually starts in adulthood; *occupational asthma* is caused by workplace exposures	*Physical exam:* reduced airflow; wheezes; tachypnea; tachycardia; pulsus paradoxus in severe exacerbations *Spirometry:* decreased FEV$_1$, PEFR, FVC *ABGs:* hypoxemia, hypocapnia usually; hypercapnia seen with respiratory failure	Wheezing: chest tightness; breathlessness; cough	*Relieve airway inflammation:* inhaled corticosteroids, oral or IV preparations may be necessary *Relieve bronchospasm:* inhaled bronchodilators, oral or IV preparations may be necessary; inhaled anticholinergics *Prevent bronchospasm:* sodium cromoglycate may be administered to prevent early and late response to allergens; environmental strategies to control allergens and irritants

(Continued)

Table 22 Etiology, Manifestations, and Treatment of Respiratory Disorders (cont'd)

Disorder/Definition	Cause	Signs	Symptoms	Treatment
Chronic bronchitis (*Age group = adults*) Cough and sputum production 3 mo per yr for 2 yr in succession *or* chronic productive cough present for half the time for 2 yr without known cause	Chronic airway irritation from inhaled substances, especially cigarette smoke	*Physical exam:* crackles and rhonchi; peripheral edema, jugular venous distention, S3 and S4 if heart failure present; increased anterior-posterior diameter and flattened diaphragms with severe obstruction *Spirometry:* decreased FEV1, PEFR, FVC *ABGs:* may see hypoxemia, hypercapnia	Productive cough; breathlessness	Promote secretion clearance; smoking cessation; bronchodilators, usually inhaled and oral; maybe corticosteroids and anticholinergics; measures to enhance secretion clearance; antibiotics for exacerbations; low-flow oxygen for hypoxemia; diuretics for heart failure; strategies to control breathlessness

(Continued)

Table 22   Etiology, Manifestations, and Treatment of Respiratory Disorders (cont'd)

Disorder/Definition	Cause	Signs	Symptoms	Treatment
Emphysema (*Age group = adults*)				
"Abnormal permanent enlargement of air-spaces distal to the terminal bronchioles accompanied by destruction of their walls and without fibrosis" (Snider, 1985)	Cigarette smoking; α_1-antitrypsin deficiency	*Physical exam:* increased anterior-posterior diameter; flattened diaphragms; decreased air movement on chest auscultation *Spirometry:* decreased FEV_1, PEFR, FVC *Other pulmonary function tests:* decreased diffusing capacity for carbon monoxide *ABGs:* hypoxemia, hypercapnia	Breathlessness	Relieve breathlessness: bronchodilators, inhaled and oral; low-flow oxygen for hypoxemia; strategies to control breathlessness; smoking cessation

(Continued)

Table 22 Etiology, Manifestations, and Treatment of Respiratory Disorders (cont'd)

Disorder/Definition	Cause	Signs	Symptoms	Treatment
Chronic obstructive pulmonary disease (COPD); may be called chronic obstructive lung disease (COLD) or chronic airflow obstruction (CAO) *(Age group = adults)*				
Airway obstruction that may be partially reversible with presence of emphysema or chronic bronchitis; may also include cystic fibrosis and other obstructive diseases	Same as chronic bronchitis and emphysema	Same as chronic bronchitis and emphysema	Same as chronic bronchitis and emphysema	Same as chronic bronchitis and emphysema
Bronchiolitis obliterans *(Age group = infants and young children)*				
Chronic obstruction of bronchioles after acute bronchiolitis	Formation of bronchiolar granulation tissue and peribronchiolar fibrosis	*Physical exam:* wheezing	Wheezing; cough; dyspnea	Steroids; surgical resection if localized

(Continued)

Table 22   Etiology, Manifestations, and Treatment of Respiratory Disorders (cont'd)

Disorder/Definition	Cause	Signs	Symptoms	Treatment
Cystic fibrosis (CF) *(Age group = neonate to adult)*				
Exocrine pancreatic insufficiency and/or chronic airway obstruction *Diagnostic criteria:* pulmonary manifestations and/or gastrointestinal manifestations and/or history of CF in immediate family and sweat chloride concentration > 60 mEq/L	Autosomal recessive genetic disorder; incidence 1:2500 whites	*Pulmonary disease:* crackles; increased anterior-posterior diameter, flattened diaphragms, clubbing of digits; bronchiectasis; colonization with *Pseudomonas* *Spirometry:* decreased FEV_1, PEFR, FVC *ABGs:* hypoxemia, hypercapnia (end stage) *Gastrointestinal disease:* meconium ileus in newborns and meconium ileus equivalent in adults; protein and fat malabsorption	*Pulmonary disease:* Productive cough; breathlessness; maybe hemoptysis; recurrent infection *Gastrointestinal disease:* frequent, foul-smelling, greasy stools *Exocrine dysfunction:* weakness, lethargy due to hyponatremia (heat prostration)	*Promote secretion clearance:* Chest physical therapy; bronchodilators; inhaled corticosteroids as needed; regular exercise *Control infection:* antibiotics, oral, inhaled, and/or IV; avoid crowds in flu season; flu vaccine *Promote nutrition:* pancreatic enzyme replacement; vitamins; dietary supplements; hydration/salt replacement if necessary

(Continued)

Table 22   Etiology, Manifestations, and Treatment of Respiratory Disorders (cont'd)

Disorder/Definition	Cause	Signs	Symptoms	Treatment
		Other exocrine gland dysfunction: sweat gland dysfunction with excessive salt loss; male infertility *Associated problems:* sinusitis; nasal polyps; diabetes; pancreatitis; biliary cirrhosis; cholelithiasis; pneumothorax; frank hemoptysis; hematemesis		*Psychosocial support:* promote self-care/independence; normalize life as much as possible; genetic counseling *Lung transplantation*

(Continued)

Table 22   Etiology, Manifestations, and Treatment of Respiratory Disorders (cont'd)

Disorder/Definition	Cause	Signs	Symptoms	Treatment
Bronchiectasis *(Age group = childhood to adult)*				
Abnormal dilation of bronchi more than 2 mm diameter from destruction of muscular and elastic tissue; can be localized or generalized	Associated with chronic bacterial infection, bronchial obstruction, congenital defects such as cystic fibrosis, Kartagener's syndrome, α1-antitrypsin deficiency	*Physical exam:* crackles; rhonchi; wheezes; sometimes clubbing; cyanosis, right ventricular failure *Spirometry:* decreased FEV1, FVC, PEFR *ABGs:* may see hypoxemia; hypercapnia	Chronic cough with purulent sputum (three layers); fever, weakness, weight loss; sometimes hemoptysis	*Promote secretion clearance:* chest physical therapy; bronchodilators; antibiotics
Bronchopulmonary dysplasia (BPD) *(Age group = infants [can be seen in adults who have had adult respiratory distress syndrome])*				
Bronchiolar metaplasia, obliteration, and cyst formation	Long-term positive-pressure ventilation with high oxygen concentrations to treat infant respiratory distress syndrome (hyaline	*Physical exam:* retractions; expiratory grunting; nasal flaring; crackles; wheezing *ABGs:* hypoxemia, hypercapnia	Cough; irritability; lethargy	Correct hypoxemia: mechanical ventilation; oxygen therapy (gradual withdrawal of both as tolerated); chest physical therapy

(Continued)

Table 22 Etiology, Manifestations, and Treatment of Respiratory Disorders (cont'd)

Disorder/Definition	Cause	Signs	Symptoms	Treatment
	membrane disease or other diseases requiring respiratory support measures)			*Relieve bronchospasm:* bronchodilators; steroids *Treat infection:* antibiotics *Supportive care:* nutritional support; developmental support
RESTRICTIVE DISORDERS				
Interstitial pulmonary fibrosis (cryptogenic fibrosing alveolitis) *(Age group = infant to adult; mean age 50–60 yr)* Chronic inflammation of the alveolar walls leading to progressive fibrosis	Unknown	*Physical exam:* finger clubbing in 40%–80% of patients; fine end inspiratory crackles (Velcro rales); tachypnea *Spirometry:* normal PEFR and FEV$_1$; decreased VC	Breathlessness; cough (may be dry or productive of scant mucoid sputum)	*Control breathlessness:* corticosteroids; immunosuppressant therapy; nursing strategies *Relieve hypoxemia:* oxygen therapy

(Continued)

Table 22   Etiology, Manifestations, and Treatment of Respiratory Disorders (cont'd)

Disorder/Definition	Cause	Signs	Symptoms	Treatment
		ABGs: Severe hypoxemia; normal or low $PaCO_2$; hypercapnia when end stage		
Coal worker's pneumoconiosis (black lung disease) *(Age group = adult)*				
Coal macules and nodules; focal emphysema and nodules and fibrosis from deposition of coal dust	Inhalation and deposition of coal dust in lung; frequently associated with bronchitis and emphysema from cigarette smoking; individual susceptibility is a factor	*Physical exam:* crackles; signs of right ventricular failure *Spirometry:* decreased VC; decreased FEV_1 and PEFR if associated bronchitis and emphysema *ABGs:* may see hypoxemia, hypercapnia	Productive cough (may see black sputum); breathlessness	*Control breathlessness:* nursing strategies; control exposures to coal dust; bronchodilators if obstruction present; oxygen for hypoxemia; diuretics for heart failure *Smoking cessation strategies* *Surveillance for TB*

(Continued)

Table 22 Etiology, Manifestations, and Treatment of Respiratory Disorders (cont'd)

Disorder/Definition	Cause	Signs	Symptoms	Treatment
Asbestosis (pulmonary parenchymal fibrosis) *(Age group = adult)*				
Pulmonary fibrosis and pleural thickening from inhalation of asbestos fibers	Inhalation of asbestos fibers; disease dependent on amount inhaled and individual response; frequently associated with bronchitis and emphysema from cigarette smoking; individual susceptibility is a factor	*Physical exam:* basilar crackles; coarse rhonchi; sometimes finger clubbing *Spirometry:* not diagnostic *ABGs:* sometimes hypoxemia and hypercapnia	Breathlessness; productive cough; chest tightness; chest pain	Relieve breathlessness: bronchodilators may be helpful; nursing strategies; oxygen for hypoxemia *Smoking cessation strategies*
Kyphoscoliosis (with chronic respiratory failure) *(Age group = adults more than 35 yr; cause of < 1% of chronic respiratory failure in adults)*				
Excessive curvature of spine (kyphosis–posterior curvature; scoliosis–lateral curvature) causing	Defect in vertebrae, connective tissue, or neuromuscular support of spinal column; one	*Physical exam:* abnormal thoracic cage; reduced breath sounds; heart failure (end stage)	Breathlessness; reduced activity tolerance; repeated respiratory infections	Surgery usually does not correct lung complication in adults *Supportive care:* avoidance of infection;

(Continued)

Table 22 Etiology, Manifestations, and Treatment of Respiratory Disorders (cont'd)

Disorder/Definition	Cause	Signs	Symptoms	Treatment
reduced lung volumes and pulmonary vascular bed, stiff chest wall, re-duced respiratory muscle strength, and hypoventi-lation	third of patients also have emphysema and bronchitis; two thirds have atelectasis	*Spirometry:* decreased VC (FEV₁ decreased in proportion to VC in patients with scoliosis curves greater than 90-100 degrees) *ABGs:* hypoxemia, hypercapnia		treatment of infection; avoidance of sedatives; oxygen for hypoxemia; mechanical ventilation for respiratory failure if necessary
NEUROMUSCULAR DISORDERS				
Myasthenia gravis (*Age group = adult*) Motor end-plate disease causing muscle weak-ness aggravated by muscle contraction	IgG autoantibody affecting skeletal muscle acetylcholine receptors	*Physical exam:* tachypnea; muscle wasting *Spirometry:* decreased VC *ABGs:* hypoxemia and hypercapnia in respiratory failure	Progressive weakness; breathlessness; decreased cough; dysphagia; difficult speech; decreased gag reflex	*Treat cause:* anticholinesterase; corticosteroids; plasmapheresis to remove IgG autoantibody *Supportive care:* prevention of infection; respiratory support as

(Continued)

Table 22 Etiology, Manifestations, and Treatment of Respiratory Disorders (cont'd)

Disorder/Definition	Cause	Signs	Symptoms	Treatment
				required; promote secretion clearance
Amyotrophic lateral sclerosis (Lou Gehrig's disease) *(Age group = adult)*				
Upper and lower motor neuron deficits causing muscle atrophy	Progressive degeneration of cortico-spinal tract neurons, brainstem, and spinal cord motor cells	*Physical exam:* peripheral muscle weakness; tachypnea; decreased diaphragmatic movement; sometimes heart failure *Spirometry:* decreased VC *ABGs:* hypoxemia and hypercapnia in respiratory failure	Limb and respiratory muscle weakness; may have muscle cramps and fasciculations: fatigue and breathlessness with exertion progressing to breathlessness at rest; decreased cough, speaking and swallowing ability, and gag reflex; may have morning headache, disturbed sleep, daytime somnolence	*Supportive care:* intermittent to continuous ventilatory support (negative-pressure body respirators); postural drainage; chest physical therapy with abdominal assist coughing; tracheal suctioning

(Continued)

Table 22   Etiology, Manifestations, and Treatment of Respiratory Disorders (cont'd)

Disorder/Definition	Cause	Signs	Symptoms	Treatment
Poliomyelitis (*Age group = any age; rare now because of vaccination; now see late denervation of muscles that were reinnervated earlier*)				
Destruction of motor neurons in anterior horn cells of spinal cord causing muscle paralysis	Viral infection	*Physical exam:* decreased chest expansion; decreased reflexes; muscle atrophy *Spirometry:* decreased VC *ABGs:* hypoxemia, hypercapnia dependent on degree of respiratory failure	Muscle paralysis; breathlessness	*Promote ventilation:* ventilatory assistance dependent on degree of paralysis; glossopharyngeal breathing *Promote secretion clearance:* same as spinal cord injuries
Myopathy (*Age group = child to adult*)				
Muscle weakness	Congenital defects; infection; diabetes mellitus; steroids; alcohol; impaired nutrition; inflammatory autoimmune disease	*Physical exam:* may see muscle atrophy and fasciculation; tachypnea; if advanced may see impaired gag reflex, decreased diaphragm-	Limb and respiratory muscle weakness; breathlessness; if extreme, difficulty speaking, coughing, and swallowing; may also	*Treat cause* *Supportive care:* speech and cough techniques; phrenic nerve pacing; mechanical ventilation

(Continued)

Table 22   Etiology, Manifestations, and Treatment of Respiratory Disorders (cont'd)

Disorder/Definition	Cause	Signs	Symptoms	Treatment
		atic excursion, and heart failure *Spirometry:* decreased VC *ABGs:* hypoxemia, hypercapnia if severe	have morning headache, difficulty sleeping, and daytime sleepiness	
Spinal Cord Injuries **High cervical injury** *(Age group = any age)*				
Injury above C3 leading to respiratory muscle paralysis	Usually traumatic; may be tumors; epidural abscess, vascular accident	*Physical exam:* apnea; decreased breath sounds; sometimes basilar rhonchi; sometimes hypertrophy of sternocleidomastoid and trapezius muscles; flaccid abdominal muscles; no diaphragmatic excursion with respiration	Inability to breathe, talk, or cough; asphyxia; dyspnea; difficulty clearing secretions	*Promote ventilation:* glossopharyngeal breathing, speech, and cough techniques; phrenic nerve pacing and/or mechanical ventilation *Promote secretion clearance:* turn every 2 hr; suctioning as necessary; bronchodilators

(Continued)

Table 22   Etiology, Manifestations, and Treatment of Respiratory Disorders (cont'd)

Disorder/Definition	Cause	Signs	Symptoms	Treatment
				for retained secretions; antibiotics for infection
Mid and low cervical injury (*Age group = any age*)				
Quadriplegia: C3–C8 lesion with paralysis of all four limbs; usually some respiratory function	Same as high cervical injury	*Physical exam:* paradoxic movement of rib cage; crackles and rhonchi with retained secretions and infection *Spirometry:* decreased VC (increased VC in supine position) *ABGs:* normal awake PaCO$_2$ to mild hypercapnia and hypoxemia	Breathlessness with retention of secretions and infection	*Promote secretion clearance:* change position every 2 hr; deep breathing exercises and incentive spirometry every 4 hr; chest physical therapy; assisted coughing; bronchodilators and bronchoscopy for retained secretions; antibiotics for infection *Increase ventilatory muscle strength:* inspiratory and expiratory muscle resistance training

(Continued)

Table 22   Etiology, Manifestations, and Treatment of Respiratory Disorders (cont'd)

Disorder/Definition	Cause	Signs	Symptoms	Treatment
Thoracic cord injury (*Age group = any age*)				
Paraplegia	Same as high cervical injury	May be same as mid and low cervical injury or less severe depending on level of injury	Same as high cervical injury	*Enhance cough effectiveness* *Enhance expiratory muscle strength*
OTHER DISORDERS				
Pulmonary embolism (*Age group = adult*)				
Partial or complete obstruction of pulmonary arteries and vasoconstriction causing increased pulmonary vascular resistance and increased right ventricular work	95% of occurrence from venous thrombosis of legs, rarely from arms, hepatic or renal veins, right atrium or ventricle (more likely with right heart failure or indwelling catheter); venous thrombosis is associated with venous stasis from immobility, right ventricular failure, and peripheral edema; thrombosis is	*Physical exam:* tachypnea; tachycardia, cyanosis; right ventricular failure; sometimes hemoptysis; crackles, dullness *Spirometry:* nondiagnostic *ABGs:* hypoxemia	Sudden onset of chest pain, breathlessness, palpitations, and sense of impending doom	*Relieve obstruction of pulmonary arteries:* anticoagulant therapy; rarely thrombolytic agents, surgical embolectomy, and inferior vena cava interruption to prevent recurrences *Supportive care:* oxygen therapy for hypoxemia; treatment of heart failure

(Continued)

Table 22   Etiology, Manifestations, and Treatment of Respiratory Disorders (cont'd)

Disorder/Definition	Cause	Signs	Symptoms	Treatment
	result of internal injury and coagulation defects			*Prevention of venous thrombosis:* low-dose anticoagulants and leg compressive devices for patients at significant risk
Spontaneous pneumothorax *(Age group = infant to adult)*				
Air in pleural space	Can be primary from rupture of subpleural bleb of unknown cause or secondary to underlying lung disease, when it can be life threatening; associated with chronic obstructive pulmonary disease, cystic fibrosis, *Pneumocystis carinii* pneumonia, bronchogenic carcinoma, tuberculosis, and neonatal respiratory distress syndrome; may occur with positive-pressure mechanical ventilation	*Physical exam:* tachycardia; cyanosis; hypotension; mediastinal shift toward opposite side; hyperresonance, distant breath sounds, decreased tactile fremitus on affected side *Spirometry* (if performed): decreased VC *ABGs:* hypoxemia; hypercapnia; tension pneumothorax may cause	Sudden onset of breathlessness, chest pain on affected side	*Removal of pleural air:* tube thoracostomy *Prevention of recurrence:* pleural instillation of sclerosing agent; thoracotomy to oversew or remove bullae *Supportive care:* oxygen, pain control

(Continued)

Table 22   Etiology, Manifestations, and Treatment of Respiratory Disorders (cont'd)

Disorder/Definition	Cause	Signs	Symptoms	Treatment
		acute respiratory failure		
Lung cancer (bronchogenic carcinoma 90% of lung cancer) *(Age group = adult)*				
Carcinoma arising from basal cells of bronchial mucosa; includes squamous cell, adeno-carcinoma, large cell, and adenosquamous cell carcinoma (small cell and non-small cell)	80%-85% of cases from cigarette smoking; other associated factors are inhalation of asbestos and other carcinogens, low dietary vitamin A, familial tendency, immunocompromise, and chronic obstructive pulmonary disease	*Physical exam:* may be normal; stridor or absent breath sounds if partial or complete obstruction of bronchus; pneumonitis or pleural effusion; may see clubbing *Spirometry:* not diagnostic *ABGs:* depend on degree of pulmonary disease	Dependent on location and whether primary or metastatic *Primary lung:* cough; sputum; hemoptysis; breathlessness; chest pain; fever *Intrathoracic extrapulmonary:* breathlessness; wheezing; chest pain; hoarseness; dysphagia; super-	*Surgical resection if possible* *Pain control* *Radiation/chemotherapy* *Psychosocial support* *Nutritional support* *Palliative control of symptoms*

(Continued)

Table 22   Etiology, Manifestations, and Treatment of Respiratory Disorders (cont'd)

Disorder/Definition	Cause	Signs	Symptoms	Treatment
			ior vena cava obstruction; cardiac symptoms *Metastases:* lymph node enlargement, central nervous system symptoms; liver enlargement and pain; bone pain; cutaneous or subcutaneous masses *Systemic symptoms:* anorexia; weight loss; weakness; neurologic symptoms	

(Continued)

Table 22 Etiology, Manifestations, and Treatment of Respiratory Disorders (cont'd)

Disorder/Definition	Cause	Signs	Symptoms	Treatment
Respiratory failure (*Age group = infant to adult*)				
Abnormal gas exchange resulting in ventilatory failure with $PaCO_2$ > 45 mm Hg and/or impaired oxygenation with PaO_2 < 60 mm Hg while breathing room air; can be acute or chronic; many home care patients have chronic respiratory failure	*Ventilatory failure:* impaired central control (Ondine's curse, cerebrovascular accident, head trauma, encephalitis, drug overdose, central apnea); impaired respiratory muscle function (neuromuscular disease, spinal cord injury); mechanical problems of lungs and chest wall (airway obstruction, obesity, kyphoscoliosis) *Impaired oxygenation:* alveolar hypoventilation (see ventilatory failure); impaired diffusion; emphysema; ventilation-perfusion mismatching; pulmonary embolism; airway	*Physical exam:* rapid, shallow breathing or decreased ineffective respirations or apnea; sometimes coma and cardiovascular collapse (see also acute respiratory failure in patient with chronic respiratory failure, below)	Breathlessness; orthopnea (see also acute respiratory failure in patient with chronic respiratory failure, below)	Hospitalization *Treat cause if known:* antibiotics for infection; chest tube for pneumothorax; anticoagulants for pulmonary embolus; adjust maintenance medications; bronchodilators; corticosteroids for acute airway obstruction *Maintain oxygenation:* increase FIO_2; intubation and mechanical ventilation if necessary *Maintain secretion clearance:* chest physical therapy; suctioning if necessary

(Continued)

Table 22   Etiology, Manifestations, and Treatment of Respiratory Disorders (cont'd)

Disorder/Definition	Cause	Signs	Symptoms	Treatment
	obstruction; right to left shunting of blood; pneumonia; atelectasis; pulmonary edema (intracardiac shunt, arteriovenous failure); reduced FIO_2; fire exposure			
Acute respiratory failure in client with chronic respiratory failure (*Age group = infant to adult*)				
Inability to maintain PaO_2 of approximately 60 mm Hg with variable $PaCO_2$ on maximal therapy	*Infection:* inflammation; excessive secretions *Acute bronchoconstriction:* allergen exposure; noxious gas inhalation *Pneumothorax* *Pulmonary embolism* *Reduction in maintenance doses of medications*	Must know what is usual for client *Physical exam:* may see increased use of accessory muscles, grunting, nasal flaring, pulsus paradoxus 15 mm Hg or more; reduced breath sounds; tachycardia	Must know what is usual for client; may see increased breathlessness, increased cough, increase or decrease in sputum production, more	See respiratory failure (above)

(Continued)

Table 22 Etiology, Manifestations, and Treatment of Respiratory Disorders (cont'd)

Disorder/Definition	Cause	Signs	Symptoms	Treatment
		(more than 130 beats/min); inability to cooperate; restlessness; increased signs of heart failure; fever *Spirometry:* client may be unable to perform; decreased FVC, FEV_1, PEFR *ABGs:* worsening PaO_2 on usual flow rate of supplemental oxygen; variable $PaCO_2$	tenacious sputum	

Turner J, McDonald G, and Larter N: *Handbook of pediatric and adult respiratory home care,* St. Louis, 1994, Mosby–Year Book, Inc.

Nursing Interventions for the Client with Acute Respiratory Tract Infection*

Effective Use of Medications

- Teach client and caregiver proper administration of prescribed medications.
- Observe for effectiveness of therapy by decreased signs and symptoms of acute infection.
- Increase frequency of inhaled bronchodilators for increased bronchospasm or wheezing.
- Check with physician about adjunctive corticosteroid therapy if client is already using maximal doses of bronchodilators or is experiencing side effects and is unable to increase the dosage sufficiently to reduce symptoms. Overuse of bronchodilators without antiinflammatory agents increases risk of death. Clients who are receiving maintenance corticosteroid therapy may need to increase the dose temporarily.
- Antipyretic drugs such as Tylenol every 4 to 6 hrs may be necessary to reduce discomfort from high fevers.
- Consider possibility of drug interactions. Antibiotics such as erythromycin decrease hepatic clearance and can cause an increase in serum levels of other drugs, such as theophylline, that are cleared by the liver. It may be necessary to obtain blood for a serum theophylline level and adjust the dose accordingly if antibiotic therapy is instituted.

Adequate Intake of Food and Fluids

- Encourage adult clients to drink approximately eight large glasses (2 qt) of liquid each day unless fluid restrictions are necessary because of heart or renal failure.
- Offer juice and water to young children and infants hourly.
- Adequate fluids are particularly important to prevent dehydration of the client is febrile.
- Frequent small meals may be indicated if a respiratory tract infection causes clients to feel more short of breath while eating.
- High-calorie food supplements may be appropriate after meals or at bedtime if clients are unable to maintain adequate dietary intake.

*Turner J, McDonald G, and Larter N: *Handbook of pediatric and adult respiratory home care*, St. Louis, 1994, Mosby-Year Book, Inc.

Adequate Oxygenation

- Clients may become hypoxemic during acute phase of respiratory tract infection.
- Monitor oxygen saturation with pulse oximeter or arterial blood gas measurement.
- Supplemental oxygen should be administered as necessary to maintain oxygen saturation at 90% or higher.
- Monitor adequacy of ventilation in clients on home ventilators. It may be necessary to adjust ventilator settings temporarily during acute infection.

Adequate Secretion Clearance

- Increase frequency of bronchial hygiene measures, such as therapeutic coughing, postural drainage with percussion, and vibration, if client is having difficulty clearing secretions.
- Review bronchial hygiene regimen with client and caregiver to be sure that techniques are appropriate and being performed effectively.
- Encourage client to take frequent deep breaths to prevent atelectasis and enhance mucociliary clearance. Incentive spirometers may motivate some clients to take deeper breaths.
- Oropharyngeal suctioning may be necessary for clients who are unable to clear secretions. It may be necessary to increase frequency of suctioning if client has tracheostomy.
- Avoid cough suppressants that dry secretions and interfere with clearance.

Relief of Breathlessness

- Above interventions may be adequate to relieve breathlessness associated with acute infection.
- May be necessary to reduce or temporarily suspend exercise programs and encourage more frequent rest periods.
- Promote strategies such as positioning and coordination of activities with breathing to help provide relief.

Infection Control

- Maintain appropriate infection control precautions.
- Respiratory secretions should be discarded properly.
- May be necessary to increase frequency of cleaning of home respiratory therapy and ventilator equipment, suction catheters, and tracheostomy tubes, particularly if secretions are thick and copious.

- Home care staff, clients, and caregivers must wash their hands carefully before and after administering treatments and providing care. Universal body substance precautions must be followed.

Provide Necessary Client Monitoring

- Increase frequency of home visits during acute phase of infection for client monitoring and support.
- Clients and caregivers may be less able to cope and may become excessively anxious at such times.
- Additional support from home care staff may mean difference between successful management at home and the need for hospitalization.
- Hospitalization may be necessary if client continues to deteriorate despite optimal home care.

Therapeutic Coughing

Therapeutic coughing is a coughing technique that may enhance clearance of secretions in clients who are weak or debilitated or who experience side effects from coughing. It should be performed as follows (Turner, 1994):

1. Sit upright with both feet firmly supported.
2. Take a few deep, relaxed breaths while sitting upright.
3. Exhale through pursed lips.
4. Inhale slowly and deeply.
5. Lean forward while producing two to three short, consecutive coughs from deep in the chest. The short cough maneuvers should be made on the same exhalation. A pillow can be held tightly against the abdomen to provide support with contraction of the muscles of the abdomen and permit a stronger cough.
6. Take a few more relaxed breaths.
7. Repeat the cough maneuver two or three times until secretions are raised.

Chest Physical Therapy

A major complication of immobility and illness is the development of retained secretions, which predisposes the client to atelectasis or pneumonia. Some clients, such as those with chronic bronchitis, bronchiectasis, cystic fibrosis, or a lung abscess, have hypersecretion of mucus and retention of sputum from chronic lung diseases. Chest physical therapy (also called chest PT or CPT) uses one or more techniques to enhance removal of secretions from the airways when deep breathing (including incentive spirometry) and coughing are ineffective.

Traditionally, chest physical therapy includes postural drainage, chest percussion, vibration, and rib shaking. Deep breathing and coughing remain important when chest physical therapy is used. Review the pulmonary rehabilitation techniques of pursed-lip and diaphragm breathing before initiating chest physical therapy. Throughout chest physical therapy, the client performs pursed-lip and diaphragm breathing to enhance relaxation, to promote gas exchange, and to prevent alveolar collapse.

The nurse works with the respiratory and physical therapists in performing chest physical therapy. Nurses may perform CPT or may coordinate it with additional treatments by other therapists. Especially with clients fed by gastric tube, the nurse works with the therapist to schedule feedings and treatments. Chest physical therapy also must be scheduled with regard to sitting in the chair, weaning trials, rest periods, and other treatments. When a physical therapist performs CPT but a respiratory therapist administers inhaled bronchodilator treatments, efforts must be coordinated to optimize both treatments (Dettenmeier, 1992).

Postural Drainage

Postural drainage (also called PD) refers to positioning of the client to facilitate gravitational drainage of secretions from various segments of the lung. The rationale for positioning is that secretions will move by gravity, instead of against it, from distal to proximal areas of the lung, where they can be coughed out. In general, the area being drained is uppermost, usually facing the ceiling. This allows the bronchus to be at a vertical or near vertical position to maximize gravitational drainage.

The positions used for PD are determined by the client's clinical status. Before performing postural drainage, the nurse must know the following:

- The client's diagnosis and clinical status, as well as his or her neurological status, cardiac status, and activity level
- The lung areas involved (as indicated by auscultation and chest x-ray film)
- The history of previous thoracic operations
- Whether the client has osteoporosis or any structural abnormalities, such as fractured ribs

The client's diagnosis often identifies the area to receive percussion, such as "right lower lobe pneumonia." Most clients do not need every postural drainage position. A common exception is a client with cystic fibrosis or some other homogenous disease. When a specific segment or lobe is involved, chest physical therapy is directed to that area, saving the nurse and the client time and energy.

Secretions usually pool in the lower and middle lung fields. In bedridden clients, the posterior areas of the lung are often involved. Postural drainage positions are modified according to the client's clinical condition (see Figure 5). However, keep in mind that altering the chest physical therapy position may decrease the effectiveness of the treatment.

The type and amount of sputum produced sometimes can be predicted on the basis of the client's diagnosis, as can be seen in the following list:

Atelectasis	Minimal sputum production
Bronchiectasis	Copious, thick, viscid sputum, often hard to expectorate.
Lung abscesses	Foul smelling, purulent, and thick secretions
Pneumonia	Thick mucus plugs

Longer periods of gravitational drainage are necessary to allow thicker secretions to move.

The client's neurological and cardiovascular status are two important factors to consider when administering postural drainage. Gravitational drainage can aggravate the condition of clients with certain conditions.

In mobile clients the upper lobes frequently do not require gravitational drainage unless certain segments are involved, since the upper lobes drain in upright individuals. The exception is the client with upper lobe tuberculosis who requires postural drainage, usually in conjunction with percussion. In addition, clients confined to bed and lying with the head of the bed flat are apt to aspirate or accumulate secretions throughout the lung fields. Frequently changing the client's position (side lying, supine, or prone with head flat and at various elevations) helps to prevent secretions from accumulating in a particular area. Precautions to consider with chest physical therapy are highlighted in Table 23.

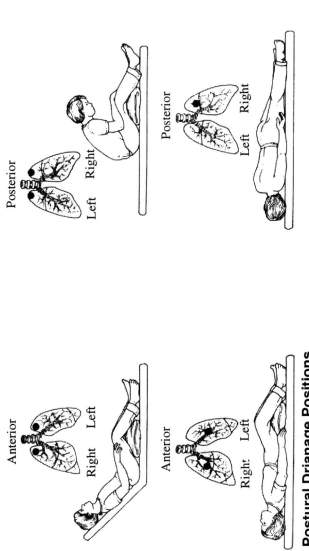

Figure 5 Postural Drianage Positions

From Thompson J et al.: *Mosby's Clinical Nursing, ed. 3*, St. Louis, 1993, Mosby-Year Book, Inc.

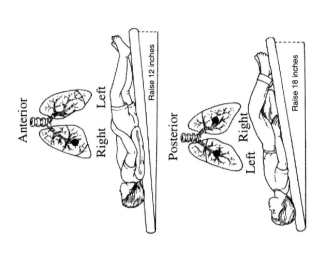

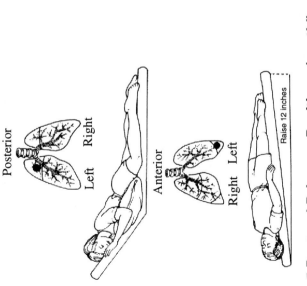

Figure 5 Postural Drainage Positions (cont'd)

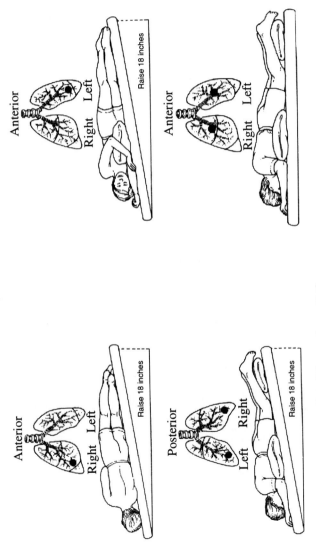

Figure 5 Postural Drianage Positions (cont'd)

Table 23   Precautions With Chest Physical Therapy

Condition	Precaution
Cardiac precautions	
Acute myocardial infarction	Head-down positions may aggravate ischemia and extend infarct.
Gastrointestinal precautions	
Gastric reflux	Use caution and perform CPT before meals. Head-down positions promote gastric reflux.
Gastric tube feedings	Use caution. Continuous feedings should be stopped 1 hour before PD, which can greatly reduce caloric intake. PD is performed before administration of intermittent feedings. Duodenal or jejunal tube feedings may continue if there is no retrograde reflux.
Neurological precautions	
Increased intracranial pressure	Head-down positions increase intracranial blood volume and intracranial pressure.
Cervical spinal cord injury with client in tongs	Altering the incline of the neck changes alignment and may aggravate injury. However, in some cases the head of the bed can be kept at its ordered level and Trendelenburg positioning of the entire bed can be used to alter the position of the lower lungs relative to the head.

(Continued)

Table 23 Precautions With Chest Physical Therapy (cont'd)

Condition	Precaution
Subarachnoid hemorrhage	Head-down positions increase cerebral blood pressure and may exacerbate bleeding.
Pulmonary precautions	
Severe dyspnea and anxiety	Head-down positions exacerbate dyspnea and anxiety; abdominal contents push up against the diaphragm, making inhalation difficult.
Bronchopulmonary fistula	Chest tubes are not an absolute contraindication to CPT; however, percussion may prevent sealing or enlarge the fistula.
Frank hemoptysis	Percussion may disrupt clots and exacerbate bleeding, resulting in pulmonary hemorrhage. Also, head-down positions increase blood return to the chest and may cause recruitment or distention of capillaries.
Flail chest	Percussion over the flail area exacerbates bruising or bleeding and may cause additional lung punctures.
Pulmonary embolism	Local consolidation is due to pulmonary embolism. Other clots, especially in the heart and central veins, may dislodge.

Dettenmeier PA: *Pulmonary nursing care*, St. Louis, 1992, Mosby-Year Book, Inc.

Percussion

Percussion is an adjunct to postural drainage. In some clients postural drainage alone moves secretions from smaller to larger airways, where they can be coughed out. Other clients require the assistance of percussion (also called cupping, tapping, or clapping) to facilitate the flow of mucus out of the lungs. Percussion is most useful in clients who produce at least 30 ml of sputum daily.

To perform percussion, the hand must be cupped as if to swim, cover the mouth, or scoop up a handful of water (see Figure 6). The fingers and thumb are held together tightly so that air cannot escape. The wrists rhythmically flex and extend as the hands alternately strike the chest. The arms are extended without locking the elbows, and the shoulders are relaxed. The whole rim of the hand touches the chest at the same time. As the hands contact the chest, an air pocket is created that sends vibrations through the chest.

Percussion creates a hollow sound and is not painful when performed properly. Some clinicians liken the sound to a horse's hooves on pavement. Flattened hands produce a slapping sound, and percussion performed with flat hands usually is painful. Some families become upset when they first see percussion, because they think the client is being beaten. Percussing the chest of the family member for a few seconds demonstrates that CPT is not painful but actually feels good.

Percussion is performed over a single thin layer of clothing such as a T-shirt or pajamas. Using thick clothing or towels dampens the vibrations, making the nurse work harder and the treatment less effective. After percussion the skin should not be reddened or bruised. The nurse should also note the following points when performing postural drainage and percussion:

Before

- Encourage fluids to promote hydration for thinner secretions.
- Perform chest physical therapy 30 to 60 minutes after use of inhaled bronchodilators.
- Use pillows to support the client and to promote relaxation in postural drainage positions; knees and hips are flexed to prevent back strain.
- Help the client into the PD position at least 5 minutes before percussion, as able.
- Avoid percussion for 2 hours after a meal to lessen the danger of vomiting. Schedule chest physical therapy at least 30 to 60

minutes before meals or bolus (intermittent) tube feedings. With continuous feedings through a gastric feeding tube, stop feedings at least 1 hour before CPT. With duodenal or jejunal continuous infusion feedings, continue feedings.

During

- Perform chest physical therapy, alternating percussion and vibration, for at least 3 to 5 minutes in each position, longer if tolerated and time permits.
- Auscultate the chest before and after CPT to evaluate the effectiveness of the treatment.
- Encourage pursed lip and diaphragm breathing during chest physical therapy. Slow, deep inhalations and exhalations are important. Air must get behind the mucus before it can be expectorated.
- Do not perform percussion over bony prominences such as the scapula, spine, or clavicles.
- Do not perform percussion over vital organs and sensitive tissue (for example, the breasts, kidneys, liver, and spleen).
- Provide rest periods and coughing breaks as needed.
- Rinse the client's mouth after sputum has been expectorated.
- At home clients usually perform CPT 2 to 4 times daily. When CPT is performed twice daily, the best times are early in the morning and before bed. If CPT is performed 4 times daily, it should be done before meals and at bedtime. Some clients perform CPT only once a day when they are feeling well and sputum production is minimal.

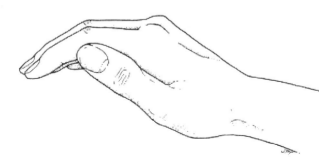

Figure 4 Hand Position for Percussion

From Beare PG and Myers JL: *Principles and practice of adult health nursing, ed. 2*, St. Louis, 1994, Mosby-Year Book, Inc.

Vibration and Rib Shaking

Vibration is another technique for enhancing gravitational drainage of secretions. Gentler than percussion, vibration is thought to increase the velocity and turbulence of exhaled air, aiding in the movement of secretions. To perform vibration, the hands are placed on the chest over the area being drained. Some clinicians fan their hands around the chest wall, whereas others place them side by side or on top of each other. The wrists are kept stiff, and the elbows are also kept stiff but not locked. Vibration is generated from the shoulder and upper arm muscles, causing a fine tremulous movement in the hands. During vibration the chest wall is gently compressed. Compression increases throughout exhalation. *Performed only during a slow, controlled exhalation,* vibration does not involve gross shaking of the client. Rib shaking, on the other hand, is very vigorous. During rib shaking the chest wall is shaken or alternately compressed and released. Vibration and rib shaking are performed 3 to 4 times, at 1-minute intervals, during percussion. Performing vibration or rib shaking during percussion aids in preventing fatigue of the nurse.

Hazards of CPT

While CPT may be beneficial, the nurse must exercise caution in its administration. The possible hazards of CPT are:

- Increase in airway resistance
- Bruising
- Fluctuations in cardiac output
- Dysrhythmias
- Fatigue
- Hypoxemia or a decrease in PaO_2
- Pain
- Rib fractures
- Wheezing

Most CPT techniques, such as coughing, are simple and can be initiated by the nurse. Timely implementation of these noninvasive techniques often can prevent the use of more aggressive invasive measures by the physician. It is important to remember that the basic nursing acts, such as teaching a client how to deep breathe and cough effectively, learned early in nursing education, are very important in maintaining or restoring the client's normal state of wellness.

Client Education: Breathing Techniques

Much of chest physical therapy demands use of pursed lip breathing, diaphragmatic breathing, or lateral chest expansion. Use the following strategies in teaching clients to perform these breathing techniques (Dettenmeier, 1992):

Pursed-Lip Breathing

- Breathe in slowly through your nose; feel your lungs fill with air.
- Purse your lips as if to whistle or kiss. Breathe out very slowly through your pursed lips. Use your lips as a gate to control air leaving the lungs.
- It should take you at least two or three times as long to breathe out as to breathe in; for example, if it takes you 2 to 3 seconds to breathe in, breathe out for at least 4 to 6 seconds.

Diaphragmatic Breathing

It often is easier to perform diaphragmatic breathing while sitting, because then your abdomen is not pushing up on your diaphragm.

- Place one hand on your abdomen just above your waist and your other hand on your upper chest. While sniffing, feel your lower hand jump; this is your diaphragm.
- Breathe in through your nose and feel your lower hand (diaphragm) push out. Your upper hand should not move.
- Breathe out through pursed lips, and feel your lower hand (diaphragm) move in.

Lateral Chest Expansion

- Place your hands on your lower ribs at your sides.
- Breathe in through your nose, and concentrate on pushing your hands out.
- Keep your shoulders still.
- Breathe out, and feel your hands move in.

Client Education:
Energy Conservation Techniques

The following tips can be shared with clients to help them conserve energy and ease breathing with exertion (Dettenmeier, 1992):

Breathing

- Use pursed-lip and diaphragmatic breathing.
- Remember to exhale on exertion.

Hygiene

- Sit in a chair or stand and rest your arms on the sink when combing your hair, brushing your teeth, or washing your face.
- In the bathtub, sit on a stool with rubber-tipped legs and use a hand-held shower or spray attachment.
- Leave the bathroom door open if humidity bothers you.
- Install safety rails in the bathtub and over the toilet to assist in moving around safely.
- Instead of drying off, wrap up in a terry cloth robe or sit on a towel, wrap a towel around your shoulders, and place a towel across your lap.

Clothing

- Dress your lower body first, because bending over impairs breathing in.
- Wear permanent-press, lightweight, loose-fitting clothing with front closures.
- Layer lightweight clothing in winter rather than wear heavy-weight clothing.
- Choose slip-on shoes instead of laced shoes and clothing with snaps instead of buttons.
- Wear clothing with elastic instead of fitted waists.

Walking

- Breathe in through your nose.
- Walk a few steps while you breathe out through pursed lips.
- Stop and breathe in through your nose.
- Continue this pattern of breathing until you reach your destination.

Climbing Stairs

- Breathe in through your nose.
- Climb a few steps while you breathe out through pursed lips.
- Stop as you breathe in through your nose; climb a few steps as you exhale.
- Continue this pattern until you reach a landing or the top of the stairs.

Kitchen

- Stock frequently used supplies at arm level.
- Use lightweight plastic dishes (or aluminum pans) instead of heavy china or ironstone.
- Use electrical appliances (mixer, blender, knife, food processor, dishwasher) in place of manual devices whenever possible.
- Sit on a stool and rest your arms on the counter or table when preparing food or washing dishes.
- Allow dishes to air dry rather than dry them by hand.
- Cook larger portions and freeze or refrigerate some for later.

Housecleaning

The key is organization.

- Push a wheeled cart with several shelves containing cleaning supplies (duster, polish, cleaning cloth, pan of water with cleaning solution) around and between rooms.
- Place items needing to be stored in another area of the house on lower shelves.
- Keep a box or basket at the top and bottom of stairs for placing items to be carried down and up, respectively. Make one trip when the box is full.
- Completely clean one side or area of the room before moving to another area. Don't waste steps.
- Finish making one side of the bed before starting the other side.
- Use a self-wringing mop if possible. Breathe out while bending forward to mop, because bending forces air from the lungs. Breathe in while standing. Lean on the mop, if necessary.
- Breathe in; while pushing vacuum, breathe out.

General

- Schedule activities requiring lots of energy early in the day.

- Perform chest therapy and take inhaled bronchodilators before heavy exertion.
- Space activities requiring lots of energy, such as mowing the lawn, shopping, and vacuuming, throughout the week.
- If possible, hire someone to perform tasks that cause excessive shortness of breath or fatigue.

Client Education: Breathing Exercises for Dyspnea

Shortness of breath or difficulty breathing, dyspnea, is a problem for clients with chronic lung diseases. Use these instructions to teach clients techniques for breathing more easily (Wilson & Thompson, 1990).

Prevention Tips

- Avoid pollutants from heavy traffic and smog. Stay away from aerosol sprays and products that produce fumes, such as paint, kerosene, and cleaning agents.
- Cold weather can trigger dyspnea. If you must go outside when it's cold, cover your mouth with a scarf or mask.
- Very dry air increases dyspnea and thickens mucus. A portable room humidifier is helpful, especially in the winter.
- Physical exertion brings on dyspnea. Learn to conserve energy by resting frequently, alternating light and heavy tasks, and minimizing movement. Instead of standing, sit. Instead of pushing or lifting objects, pull.
- Be creative in managing tasks—for example, a cart or child's wagon can be used to haul groceries, and wheels can be installed on furniture that is frequently moved.
- Breathe out slowly through pursed lips for 6 seconds (count one 100, two 100, three 100, four 100, five 100, six 100.)

Abdominal Breathing

Abdominal breathing will also slow down breathing to make it more effective. It also helps relax the entire body before sleeping.

- Lie on your back in a comfortable position with a pillow under your head. Place another pillow under your knees to help relax your abdomen.
- Rest one hand on your abdomen just below your rib cage. Rest the other hand on your chest.
- Slowly breathe in and out through your nose using your abdominal muscles. The hand resting on your abdomen will

rise when you breathe in and fall when you breathe out. The hand on your chest should be almost still.

Client Education: Using Oxygen at Home

The idea of using oxygen therapy at home sounds frightening to some clients. It sounds uncomfortable, complicated, and confusing. It also sounds dangerous. Use the following instructions when teaching the uninitiated client how to use and take care of oxygen equipment:

Your doctor has prescribed extra oxygen at a flow rate of ___ liters per minute for ___ hours every day. The medical supply company will show you how to set the flow rate and how to care for the equipment. Keep the supplier's phone number handy so that you can call if the system doesn't work properly.

You will be using a liquid oxygen unit, an oxygen tank, or an oxygen concentrator. You will breathe the oxygen through either a mask or a nasal cannula (two short prongs that fit just inside your nostrils). The system will also have a humidifier to warm and moisturize the oxygen.

It's a good idea to also have a small portable oxygen tank for an emergency backup system in case of power failure.

Here are some general guidelines and safety tips for using oxygen equipment (Wilson, 1990).

General Guidelines

- Always keep your oxygen flow rate where your doctor prescribes.
- Sometimes it's hard to tell whether oxygen is flowing through the tubes. If you have doubts, check to be sure that the system is turned on and there are no kinks in the tubing. If you still aren't sure, place the nasal cannula in a glass of water with the prongs up and watch for bubbles. (Always shake the water off before inserting the cannula into your nostrils.) If no bubbles appear, oxygen is not flowing through the tubes and you need to call the supplier.
- Each time before using oxygen, check the humidifier bottle. If it's near the fill line, empty the bottle and refill it with sterile or bottled water.
- Even with the humidifier, oxygen can dry the inside of your nose. A water-soluble lubricant (such as K-Y Jelly) helps ease dryness and cracking. Don't use petroleum-based products like Vaseline because they will make the dryness worse.

- To avoid running out of oxygen, reorder a new supply when the register reads 1/4 full—2 or 3 days before a new tank is needed.

Safety Precautions

- Keep the oxygen unit away from open flames and heat. This includes smoking— don't smoke and don't allow others to smoke around you. If you have a gas stove, gas space heater, or kerosene heater or lamp, stay out of the room while it's on.
- To prevent leakage, always keep the oxygen system upright, and make sure the system is turned off when not in use. Don't place carpets, bed clothes, or furniture over the tubing, since this may cause a leak.
- Keep an all-purpose fire extinguisher close by.
- If a fire should occur, turn off the oxygen and leave the house at once.
- Notify the local fire department that you have oxygen in the house. In most areas, the fire department offers free safety inspections, which can help make your home even safer for using oxygen.

Call Your Doctor Immediately If:

- Your breathing is difficult, irregular, shallow, or slow.
- You become restless or anxious.
- You are tired, drowsy, or have trouble waking up.
- You have a persistent headache.
- Your speech becomes slurred, you can't concentrate, or you feel confused.
- Your fingernails or lips are bluish.

These symptoms may arise when you are not getting enough oxygen or when you are getting too much oxygen. Only your doctor can determine how much oxygen you need. Therefore you must never change the flow rate without instructions from your doctor.

Chronic Renal Failure

Chronic renal failure (CRF) results from a variety of disorders and is characterized by progressive, irreversible damage to the nephrons and glomeruli. Recurrent kidney infection and/or vascular damage from diabetes or hypertension can lead to scarring of the renal tissue and are but a few of the potential causes of CRF. It may also result from unresolved acute renal failure (ARF). Renal damage may be diffuse or limited to only one kidney. The renal parenchyma is primarily affected. Regardless of the cause, the result is gradually decreasing glomerular filtration rate, tubular function, and reabsorptive capability, leading to dysfunction in fluid and electrolyte control, acid-base disturbance, and systemic problems. Generally, a gradual progression toward uremia occurs. Dialysis becomes necessary as renal function diminishes (Beare & Myers, 1994).

Table 24 summarizes key points to remember in caring for the client with chronic renal failure.

Table 24   Guidelines for Care of Clients with Chronic Renal Failure

Do's	Don'ts
If blood needs to be drawn, use the nonvascular access limb.	Do not use vascular access limb for blood pressure or venipuncture.
Use of glucose meter for determining blood glucose levels is more accurate.	Do not check urine samples of a diabetic client for glucose; diminished renal function renders the procedure useless.
Use concentrated glucose (sugar, candy bar, soft drinks) to treat hypoglycemia in a diabetic renal client.	Do not give orange juice to a hypoglycemic diabetic renal client; the potassium could be lethal.

(Continued)

Table 24   Guidelines for Care of Client with Chronic Renal Failure (cont'd)

Do's	Don'ts
Encourage use of various spices such as onion powder, garlic powder, Mrs. Dash, and so on to spice up food without adding salt.	Permit no salt substitutes; they substitute potassium chloride for sodium chloride.
Always do a multipositional blood pressure assessment (lying to sitting to standing).	Never accept a lying (supine) hypertensive blood pressure reading without following up with a sitting/standing assessment.
Assess vascular access function by listening for bruit or feeling for thrill as evidence the access is patent.	Never occlude the vascular access with constrictive clothing or B/P cuff; remind client not to carry heavy objects on the arm.
Do encourage the client to assume as much responsibility for self-care as possible.	Do not encourage dependency and complacency, as these contribute to decreased quality and quantity of life.
Do encourage the client to follow the prescribed regimen of diet, medications, and dialysis (if applicable).	Remind client that noncompliance can be very uncomfortable and lead to death in a renal client.

Modified from Martinson I and Widmer J, eds: *Home health care nursing*, Philadelphia, 1989, WB Saunders Co.

Peritoneal Dialysis

There are primarily two types of home peritoneal dialysis. The first is continuous ambulatory peritoneal dialysis. This type of dialysis involves 24-hour dialysis in which fluid is instilled into the peritoneal cavity, allowed to remain for a period of 4 to 6 hours, and then drained out of the peritoneal cavity. This procedure uses a special plastic container and connecting devices that are designed to be attached to a special catheter, surgically implanted through the abdomen into the peritoneal cavity.

The second type is continuous cycler peritoneal dialysis. This type of dialysis is designed to be used at home while the client sleeps and is an 8- to 10-hour process. The cycler machine is connected to the implanted catheter, and it continuously fills and drains the dialysate from the abdominal cavity.

These two types of dialysis work on the same principle. Dialyzing solution is infused into the peritoneal cavity. It is left in the cavity where the peritoneum is able to act as a dialyzing membrane, and wastes pass across it into the solution in the cavity. After a specified time the solution is drained from the cavity and new solution instilled.

Short-Term Goals

- The client will understand and demonstrate the procedures needed to carry out home peritoneal dialysis.
- The client will understand the physiology of peritoneal dialysis.
- The client will understand diet and fluid restrictions.
- All equipment and supplies will be available for the procedure.

Long-Term Goals

- The client will be able to carry out the procedure without complications.
- The procedure will be incorporated into the client's lifestyle with the least amount of restrictions possible.

Nursing Assessment Factors

Health Management Pattern

The client or caregiver must have a place to do the exchanges and must be able to understand the procedure and the need for meticulous cleanliness to prevent peritonitis.

Nutrition-Metabolic Pattern

Because continuous dialysis regulates the client's fluid balance and metabolic environment on a 24-hour basis, the client may be able to eat a normal diet and have only modest fluid restrictions.

Elimination

Elimination of fluid and wastes is done through the dialysate.

Activity and Exercise

There are no restrictions on activities because of the peritoneal dialysis, but activities should be discussed with the client's physician.

Sexuality-Reproductive Pattern

Many persons on dialysis continue to have an active sexual life; in some cases peritoneal dialysis may result in increased sexual activity, because the person is less tired or irritable; some persons have diminished sexual desire because of the kidney disease; dialysis affects each person differently, so concerns about sexuality must be addressed individually.

Implementation

The client must be instructed in the procedure for the continuous peritoneal dialysis (Beare & Myers, 1994):

1. In a clean environment, using sterile technique, a plastic bag of sterile dialysate is attached to the catheter that enters the peritoneal cavity.
2. The bag is raised to shoulder level or higher.
3. The roller clamp on the tubing from the bag is opened, allowing the dialysate solution to run into the peritoneal cavity; gravity pulls the solution into the abdominal cavity.
4. Once the plastic bag is empty, the roller clamp is closed, and the bag is rolled up and placed under the clothing or in a carrying pouch; this part of the procedure takes 7 to 10 minutes.

5. The client can then go about normal activities with the dialysate solution in the peritoneal cavity.

6. When the specified time is up, usually 4 or 6 hours during the day and 8 hours at night, the client unrolls the plastic bag and lowers it to a level below the abdominal cavity; then the roller clamp is opened, allowing gravity to drain the fluid out of the abdominal cavity back into the original bag; this may take 20 to 35 minutes.

7. The bag and used dialysate solution are discarded.

8. A new bag of solution is attached, and the process is started over; each "exchange"—which includes the time it takes to drain the solution from the abdominal cavity, attach a new bag using sterile technique, and fill the abdominal cavity—may take 30 to 45 minutes.

9. Instructions in the signs and symptoms of peritonitis and fluid and electrolyte balance should also be given.

10. Monitoring the client's fluid and electrolyte balance must be done on an ongoing basis; the client is taught to monitor fluid status by recording daily weight and blood pressure and glucose concentration of dialysate readings; there may be some electrolyte restrictions such as sodium, potassium, or phosphorus.

11. Dietary restrictions and requirements must be compatible with the orders of the physician; the client may need protein supplements because of the loss of protein through dialysis.

12. Clients who will be using continuous cycler peritoneal dialysis will need instruction about the cycler machine; the machine is usually set to run 8 to 10 hours while the client sleeps; this machine is set up with enough dialysate to accommodate the number of prescribed exchanges; the catheter is attached to the tubing, and the dialysate is continuously cycled into and out of the peritoneal cavity throughout the night until all the exchanges have been completed.

13. All instructions given for care must be verified.

14. The client must be instructed where to get follow-up medical care, where to get dialysis supplies, and whom to contact in case of an emergency.

15. Document all activities related to client education, ability of the client to demonstrate and manage the procedure independently, and ability of the client to tolerate the procedure.

Stroke Rehabilitation

Stroke rehabilitation nursing focuses on the comprehensive management of the stroke survivor's environment and the transfer of responsibility for care back to the client as recovery occurs. Clients learn lifelong strategies for coping with deficits and gain new control over their changed lives. The role of the nurse remains important on the rehabilitation team; nurses provide the case management among the many professionals and family members who make up the treatment group.

Nurses empower stroke survivors to take charge of their own lives. This requires ongoing assessment, team planning, and integration of care into a more normal, less institutional form. Successful nursing interventions allow the team to function optimally and the client to become as highly functional as possible.

One of the challenges in discussing the needs of stroke clients is that this is a diverse population. Stroke survivors may be young or old, minimally or severely impaired, and employed or unemployed and may have many or few family and community resources upon which to draw. These factors will have a major influence on the type and amount of assistance needed in the community.

The majority of stroke survivors sustain some residual disability. The type of assistance needed can vary from minimal help to nearly total care. The nurse can facilitate the client's reintegration into the community by assessing the client and family resources and needs and necessary support services. Medicare will subsidize visits for skilled care ordered by a physician, for a limited time. Skilled care may include physical therapy and nursing care required to administer intravenous feedings, to assess a significant change in health status, to manage tubes and catheters, and to educate client and family about equipment, medications, or procedures. In some cases, help is needed to perform ADL such as bathing, dressing, feeding, and monitoring blood pressure and medications. These activities can be performed by a home health aide and may not be subsidized by Medicare.

Stroke clients are especially vulnerable after they leave the acute care hospital or rehabilitation setting. About 10% of stroke clients admitted to emergency rooms are returned directly home without admission. An unknown number of people who suffer strokes are never seen in the acute care setting but are discovered by nurses or family members when they visit the client in the home. Thus home-dwelling stroke survivors have a variety of problems. The disabilities caused by stroke (e.g., paralysis and paresis, aphasia, dysphagia, ataxia, perceptual and behavioral deficiencies)—when added to premorbid deconditioning and chronic diseases such as diabetes, hypertension, arthritis, and cardiac disease—can severely limit activity.

Active and passive range-of-motion exercises, transfer techniques, walking, and use of bathroom decrease, and sometimes cease, after discharge.

Immobility leaves the client vulnerable to skin breakdown, decreased cardiac output and stroke volume, and increased risk for pneumonia. Inability to toilet may easily lead to reduced fluid and food intake, causing fluid and electrolyte imbalances, weight changes, malnutrition, stool impaction, and loss of bone mass. Concurrently, the stroke survivor has increasing difficulty remaining motivated to do the exercises that maintain function. The stroke survivor becomes less socially active and mobile. Social isolation causes decreased stimulation and deteriorating mental health.

Caregiver role strain (secondary to change in role, dependency needs of stroke survivor, social isolation, and physical and mental fatigue) is a prominent feature of long-term care, especially in the home. Caregivers often do not know the techniques that would help to activate and motivate the stroke survivor, although they may have been exposed to the concept at some time in the acute recovery process. Of the many reasons for this deficiency, the most prominent are reduced duration of stay in the hospital or rehabilitation facility, with less time to learn techniques, and the lack of coordinated home care services.

Care of the disabled is fragmented and often unavailable to stroke survivors and their families at home. Nurses note that the decline is especially evident in long-term care for clients who no longer receive outpatient therapies. After daily therapies are discontinued because the stroke survivor is no longer improving in function, caregivers (informal and formal) and stroke survivors themselves cease exercise and decrease mobility. Rather than maintaining the level of function they have achieved, they begin to lose the gain and enter a "sine wave" pattern of deconditioning, acute illness (usually pneumonia and decubitus ulcers), hospitalization, reinitiation of therapies, cessation of therapy because of "plateau" patterns, and acute illness. This cycle is costly in both human and financial terms.

Coordination of services in the home after hospital discharge can increase and maintain a client's functional level, can result in greater client and family satisfaction, and can require less use of acute care hospitals and nursing homes. Home health services need not be long term to be effective. Only a short period of supportive services is needed to teach the client and family how to care for themselves. Nurses carry a heavy responsibility to coordinate and ensure continuity of care (Barker, 1994).

Nutritional Considerations

Brain injury causes changes in metabolism and metabolic needs; central brain mechanisms of hunger, appetite, thirst, and satiety; ability to attend to nutritional needs; mechanics of chewing and swallowing; and the ability to shop for and prepare food independently. Stroke survivors may have all of these problems, a combination of some, or none, but they are generally at high risk for changes in nutritional status. The degree of hypermetabolic state is usually related to the degree of severity of the stroke. In the acute stage, the nurse may need to use tube feedings or total parenteral nutrition (TPN) to meet the increased metabolic need. Usual practice dictates discontinuing them at the earliest possible time.

As the stroke survivor recovers and the illness becomes more chronic, the client may develop mood disorders that affect eating patterns, social and role changes that interfere with normal eating, and long-term chewing, swallowing, and other motor deficits that make eating hazardous and unsatisfying. Stroke survivors may excessively lose or gain weight.

The importance of early assessment of ability to chew and swallow cannot be overemphasized. Dysphagia, often associated with dysarthria, can be very subtle.

RDA guidelines should serve as a basis for developing nutritional prescriptions, but the metabolic changes associated with chronic illness and stroke, in particular, may greatly change the total nutritional needs. Malnutrition and dehydration are common in the elderly stroke population. In addition to nutritional barriers, mobility problems further complicate the picture.

A nutritional assessment should be performed following the guidelines included earlier in this book. In addition, a neurologic assessment is needed to assess the client's ability to chew, swallow, gag, taste, and smell food as well as to assess coordination, mental status, neglect or inattention deficits, and perceptual and sensory deficits (Barker, 1994).

Geriatric Considerations

The needs of geriatric stroke survivors are similar to those of all other neurologically impaired elderly. The limitations in ADL and IADL imposed by the stroke may be intensified by preexisting conditions such as musculoskeletal problems, dementia, or mental health problems.

Although all stroke survivors face the challenges of lifelong exercise and self-therapy to maintain function, the elderly have far greater difficulty with preventive *deconditioning*. Deconditioning affects several body systems. It is a common phenomenon among elderly stroke survivors, usually causing increased dependency. Caregiver stress and spousal and intergeneration conflict can become evident as dependency increases.

Some of the *ethical dilemmas* regarding elderly stroke survivors include rights of the stroke survivor to choose placement, do-not-resuscitate (DNR) and quality of life decisions, competency problems, control of assets, suicide decisions (not eating, lethal prescriptions), and family roles in caregiving. At all levels of care nurses are involved in these dilemmas. Nurses should carefully consider their own values and ethics in preparation for providing a helping relationship and interventions (Barker, 1994).

Behavioral, Psychologic, and Cognitive Problems

Stroke survivors suffer neurobehavioral deficits that are a direct result of the neurologic damage or dysfunction caused by the ischemic event. The behavior seen is influenced by three major variables: (1) the premorbid psychologic profile, (2) the psychologic response to the deficits and situation surrounding the stroke event, and (3) the result of damage to various areas of the physical brain.

Confusional States and Delirium

The global response of the brain to injury includes confusional states and delirium, which reflect disordered attention. Usually, these clients have *acutely* altered sensorium, with poor recent memory, poor concentration, inability to attend, and possibly delusions, hallucinations, or frank delirium. The elderly are particularly at risk for confusional states because of translocation deficits when they are suddenly moved from home to hospital.

The confusional episodes from stroke and/or hospitalization usually resolve without treatment. However, nurses must be alert to the fact that medications can cause confusional states, and, more seriously, that combinations of brain ischemia, translocation syndromes in the elderly, and medication changes can cause devastating and frightening confusional states. The behavior seen may be paranoid responses, combative behavior with fearful components, withdrawal, excessive compliance, or psychotic symptomatology. Restraint often aggravates the behavior and is unsafe and unsuccessful. Nurses should seek the underlying cause of the problem and use alternate methods for containing the behavior until it is no longer present.

Depression and Anxiety

Some researchers suggest that stroke survivors suffer more depression than other individuals with comparable disabilities, and others suggest that these symptoms can impede the recovery process. We still know relatively little about depression in stroke clients because of the confounding problems of cognitive impairment and aphasias, which render these clients unable to express their feelings appropriately.

Depression and anxiety states clearly do occur in stroke survivors with deficits in either hemisphere, but they are difficult to detect and to treat.

Within the last decade, we have learned that depression and anxiety may have different patterns of appearance during the stroke recovery period and that some clients respond to antidepressants and other psychoactive medications. In fact, researchers have proposed that early depression has a physiologic basis that is responsive to treatment, and if the depression is avoided, the client will experience more functional gain throughout the total recovery period (Barker, 1994).

Factors to Consider When Assessing Coping in Stroke Survivors[*]

- What losses has the client experienced due to the stroke?
- Has the client experienced other recent losses in his or her life?

[*]Bronstein KS, Popovich JM, and Stewart-Amidei C: *Promoting stroke recovery: A research-based approach for nurses*, St. Louis, 1991, Mosby-Year Book, Inc.

- How does the client and family appraise their situation (primary, secondary)?
- Does the client have deficits that interfere with appraisal of his or her situation?
- What adaptive tasks does the client have to accomplish?
- What goals do the client and family have?
- Are goals of the client and family consistent with one another's?
- How did the client cope before the stroke?
- How did the family cope before the stroke?
- Are the client's coping strategies enabling him or her to manage stressors effectively?
- Are the family's coping strategies effective?
- What are the sources of hope for the client and family?

Background/Personal

- What was the client's premorbid lifestyle?
- What strengths do the client and family exhibit?
- What weaknesses do the client and family exhibit?
- What are the client's and family's values and beliefs?
- What is the control orientation of the client and family?
- What are the client's demographic characteristics (age, sex, cultural background, education level, employment status, socioeconomic status, occupation)?
- What is the likelihood that the client will resume prestroke roles in family, school, and employment?

Illness-Related Factors

- Was the stroke onset sudden or gradual?
- How recently did the stroke occur?
- In what part of the brain is the lesion located?
- How extensive is the stroke lesion?
- What was the cause of the stroke?
- Is the client at high risk for recurrence?
- Does the client have concomitant acute or chronic illnesses?
- What cognitive/perceptual deficits are present that may impair coping?
- What are the type and severity of the client's functional limitations?

Environmental Factors

- Does/will the client receive rehabilitative care?
- What is the extent and level of social support from family and friends?

- What material resources are available (money, equipment, place for discharge)?
- Will the client require a caregiver? If so, who?

Variables Considered Determinants of Functional Outcome in Stroke Survivors[*]

Intrinsic Characteristics of the Client

- Demographic: age, sex, race, and marital status
- Precise neurologic deficit:
  - Motor (hemiparesis, bilateral motor deficit, no motor deficit): degree of spasticity
  - Sensory (hemisensory deficit or other)
  - Hemianopia
  - Speech problems (dysphasia, dysarthria)
  - Organic cognitive deficits
  - Other (e.g., cerebellar ataxia, cranial nerve palsies)
- Etiology of stroke (atherothrombotic brain infarct, hemorrhage)
- Comorbid processes (concurrent medical conditions that may affect survival or functional abilities)
- Psychosocial factors (premorbid personality, usual socialization patterns, affective state, and others)
- Educational level and other skills
- Vocational status
- Financial assets

Extrinsic Characteristics of the Client's Environment

- Family constellation or significant others
- Physical environment of home
- Type of community (physical environment, resources, attitudes)
- Services available (medical, rehabilitative, ongoing)

*Barnett HJ, Mohr JP, Stein BM, and Yatsu FM: *Stroke: Pathophysiology, diagnosis, and management*, New York, 1986, Churchill Livingstone, Inc., p. 1260.

Assisting the Client to Live Independently

Emergency Alerting Services

Emergency alerting services are set up to send an alert, via an electronic device or other signal, to someone outside the home that the stroke survivor needs help. This alert sets into motion a preplanned system that ensures an emergency response. These services are especially useful for people with impaired mobility who spend a lot of time at home alone and find security in knowing they can get help in an emergency. Services are usually operated around the clock, 24 hours a day, and may be operated by a variety of companies, agencies, and hospitals. The signal may be initiated by an electronic device worn by the client who is alone. When the client is in trouble, a signal is transmitted to a switchboard operator, who then seeks help. Another alerting service, the Postal Alert, was developed by the U.S. Postal Service and alerts the carrier by a red sticker on the mailbox. If mail is not picked up, the carrier will notify an appropriate agency or service to intervene (National Stroke Association, 1989).

Meals and Transportation

Meals and transportation may be provided to assist stroke survivors whose nutritional status may be compromised or those who need transportation to health care or community events. These services may be arranged on a regular or sporadic basis to enable the client to be more independent and/or to assist him or her when family or friends are not able. Meals may be provided in a congregate setting or through home delivery. Sponsored by the Title III nutrition program of the Older Americans Act, congregate meals are available for low-income elderly stroke survivors at centrally located senior centers, public agencies, schools, or churches.

Another program also sponsored by Title III is Meals on Wheels. This program delivers a nutritionally balanced, hot noon meal and sometimes cold food for supper or breakfast the next day, to homebound elderly persons age 60 years and older.

Special accommodations for transportation may be provided by the local public transit system or by specific agencies.

Equipment and Supplies

In many cases, equipment and supplies used by the stroke client may be paid for by insurance. Medicare, Medicaid, and private insurers may pay partial or total costs, if there is a prescription from the physician; however, the amount of coverage varies, depending on the policy. The nurse can assist the client in getting prescriptions for supplies and equipment before discharge to maximize insurance coverage; he or she may also direct the stroke client to specific suppliers who are competitively priced. Figure 7 shows some of the equipment that is commonly used.

Stroke Clubs and Stroke Support Groups

Stroke clubs and stroke support groups help stroke survivors and families to get educational information, to share experiences, and to get support. Sponsored by the National Easter Seals Society, the American Heart Association, or local hospitals, stroke clubs provide social and educational opportunities in a positive supportive environment where members share experiences and resources.

In contrast, a stroke support group is a group counseling program for stroke survivors, families, and caregivers (National Stroke Association, 1989). Meetings are informal but structured and provide educational information, support for emotional needs, and assistance with resolving personal concerns. Meetings are coordinated and run by a professional, often a rehabilitation expert.

Organizations for Information and Referral

In addition to providing written information, organizations provide referrals and act as resources for stroke survivors, families, and health care professionals interested in stroke clients. By belonging to professional organizations, health care professionals have opportunities to access the most current information about stroke care and for professional development. Membership fees and donations are an important source of funding and help organizations continue to provide community services to stroke survivors and families.

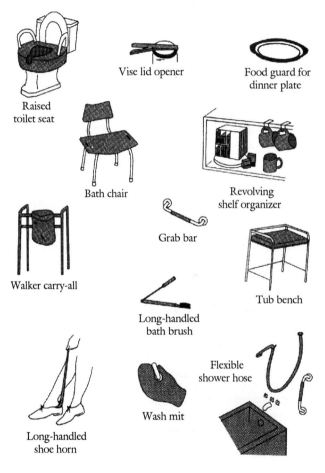

Raised toilet seat

Vise lid opener

Food guard for dinner plate

Bath chair

Revolving shelf organizer

Walker carry-all

Grab bar

Tub bench

Long-handled bath brush

Long-handled shoe horn

Wash mit

Flexible shower hose

Figure 7 Equipment Commonly Used by Stroke Clients

Bronstein KS, Popovich JM, and Stewart-Amidei C: *Promoting stroke recovery: A research-based approach for nurses*, St. Louis, 1991, Mosby-Year Book, Inc.

Acquired Immune Deficiency Syndrome

When assessing clients with AIDS, the goals of home care should be directed toward the following (Rice, 1992):

- Treating the disease and symptoms
- Preventing exacerbations of the disease (restoration and maintenance)
- Instructing clients and families regarding management of health care needs at home
- Anticipating and planning for any assistance the client may require in performing activities of daily living (ADL)
- Providing for the psychosocial and spiritual needs of the client and family

During the first visit, home health nurses should develop a plan of care based on client and family needs. An ongoing nutritional and physical assessment as well as an in-depth interview will provide clues to the appropriate interventions for clients with AIDS.

Interviewing Clients With Aids and Their Families for Assessment of Initial Needs

- What are the client's living arrangements?
- Are there family members or a lover or significant other who can assist with client care as needed?
- If the client requires home intravenous therapy, is there someone in the household willing to assist with this care?
- Who cooks and prepares the meals? (Would a referral to the registered dietitian be helpful?)
- What are the client's finances in terms of getting needed medical supplies? (Does the client need the help of a social worker?)
- Does the client have transportation to the grocery store or doctor, and is there someone who can assist with this as needed?
- Does the client need help with ADL? (Would a home health aide be helpful?)
- What does the client and the family know about AIDS, and do they have any questions about AIDS or transmission of AIDS?

■ What are the client's and family's wishes with respect to aggressive medical therapy should the client no longer be able to make decisions? Does the client have a living will, durable power of attorney, or health care proxy? (Is the situation appropriate for hospice?)

Important Topics for Client Education

- Disease process and mechanisms of transmission of HIV
- Infection control
- Medication regimen (purpose, action, dosage, side effects, methods of administration)
- Signs and symptoms of respiratory infection
- Diet
- Mouth care
- Skin care
- Safe sex
- Issues related to death and dying

Indicator Disease or Opportunistic Infections Common to Aids

Bacterial

- *Mycobacterium avium intracellulare,* MAI (disseminated)
- *Mycobacterium tuberculosis* (extrapulmonary)
- Recurrent nontyphoid salmonella septicemia (HIV positive)

Cancers

- Kaposi's sarcoma (any age if the client is HIV positive or if < 60 years old with unknown HIV status)
- Non-Hodgkin's lymphoma of B cell (HIV positive)
- Primary central nervous system lymphoma

Fungal

- Candidiasis (esophagus, trachea, bronchi, or lungs)
- Cryptococcus (extrapulmonary, typically meningitis)

Protozoal

- Cryptosporidiosis (with diarrhea longer than 1 month)
- *Pneumocystis carinii* pneumonia
- Toxoplasmosis of the brain (affecting a client > 1 month old)

Other

- Cytomegalovirus (other than liver, spleen, or lymph nodes in a client > 1 month old)
- Herpes simplex
- HIV encephalopathy (HIV dementia, AIDS dementia, or subacute encephalitis due to HIV disease—if client HIV positive)
- HIV wasting syndrome ("slime disease"—if client HIV positive)
- Lymphoid interstitial pneumonia and/or pulmonary lymphoid
- Hyperplasia in a client > 1 month old.

Infection Control Considerations*

The infection control guidelines below for persons with acquired immune deficiency syndrome (AIDS) and their caregivers are based on Centers for Disease Control (CDC) recommendations and epidemiologic data (Hughes, Marlin, & Franks, 1987). Universal precautions should be followed. The reader should refer back to the section on infection control on pages 151 to 163.

Pregnant Caregivers and AIDS

Women who are pregnant or who may be pregnant should be excused from providing direct care to a person with AIDS. The rationale for this policy is that persons with AIDS are prone to two viruses—cytomegalovirus and herpes virus—that have been known to cause serious birth defects and/or spontaneous abortions (miscarriages). Although the infection control guidelines discussed earlier would prevent caregivers from acquiring these infections if followed, the serious, harmful effects to the fetus of these viruses require particular caution. Further support for this position is found in the restriction of pregnant women from other potential occupational exposures, such as radiation therapy, that pose a threat to the fetus.

Durable Medical Equipment and AIDS

The management and cleaning of durable medical equipment (DME) is an issue of particular concern for home health care

*From Hughes A, Marlin J, and Franks P: *AIDS home care and hospice manual,* VNA of San Fransisco, 1987, AIDS Home Care and Hospice Program.

providers caring for persons with AIDS. The CDC has issued no specific guidelines for the provision or cleaning of DME used in the home of a person with AIDS. However, the CDC has recommended the use of a 10% bleach solution wipedown of *soiled* DME that cannot be sterilized by ethyl oxide or autoclaved. Most DME used at home for clients with AIDS (hospital beds, commodes, walkers, wheelchairs) cannot be autoclaved or sterilized.

San Francisco vendors who were surveyed reported that before DME is returned to the supplier, the DME is expected first to be cleaned by usual cleaning methods (using household detergents with hot water following the removal of any surface debris). The DME is then labelled "AIDS." The supplier disinfects it with a 10% bleach solution. After disinfection the DME is returned to the inventory for general circulation—*its use is not restricted to AIDS clients.*

Alzheimer's Disease

Alzheimer's disease is the most common of the neurodegenerative diseases. Although the etiology is unknown, possible causes include environmental, hereditary, and immunologic factors. The degeneration occurs in the cerebral cortex, with cortical atrophy and loss of neurons (Hogstel, 1992).

Clinical manifestations occur in three stages with some areas of overlap (see the following list). Stage one symptoms, which may last for a period of 2 to 4 years, include some memory loss, forgetfulness, and absentmindedness. The person may also experience time and spatial disorientation, decreased ability to concentrate, mistakes in judgment, changes in affect, and lack of spontaneity. In addition, there may be disturbances of perception, carelessness, delusions of persecution, muscle twitching, and seizure activity. The changes are subtle and may go unrecognized or be downplayed. Clients often become depressed during this stage when they realize that something is wrong with them (Hogstel, 1992).

The disorder is more frequently diagnosed in stage two as symptoms grow progressively worse and are more difficult to conceal. In this stage, which may extend over a longer period of time than stage one, clinical manifestations include increasing forgetfulness of both recent and remote events and intellectual changes such as inability to calculate (acalculia), to read (alexia), and to write (agraphia). Personality and behavioral changes also occur, as evidenced by increasing withdrawal and loss of socially acceptable behaviors. These changes are complicated by agnosia (inability of the client to attach meaning to sensory impressions), astereognosis (inability to recognize objects by touch), and auditory agnosia (inability to recognize familiar sounds or words), which affects comprehension. Restlessness, wandering, and sleep disorders also occur during this stage. Important papers and personal possessions are misplaced, bills go unpaid, and personal hygiene is neglected. There is an element of paranoia in that families are accused of taking papers or possessions and neighbors are accused of meddling if they offer assistance. Stage two is probably most difficult for families because of the progressive inability of the client to function and the increasing demands on family members' time and energy.

The third stage usually lasts no longer than a year and results in death, frequently as a result of aspiration pneumonia. In this stage the severity of both mental and physical symptoms has increased. The client loses the ability to perform self-care activities, no longer recognizes family members, and has lost the ability to communicate in a meaningful way with others. A decrease in appetite leads to emaciation and increased muscular weakness, and the client becomes helpless and bedridden.

Stages of Alzheimer's Disease*

Symptoms of Stage One

- Memory loss
- Time disorientation
- Spatial disorientation
- Affect changes
- Mistakes in judgment
- Absentmindedness
- Decreased concentration abilities
- Lack of spontaneity
- Perceptual disturbances
- Carelessness in actions
- Transitory delusions of persecution
- Epileptiform seizures
- Muscular twitchings

Symptoms of Stage Two

- Forgetfulness of recent and remote events
- Increased inability to comprehend
- Complete disorientation
- Restlessness at night
- Increased aphasia
- Agnosia
- Astereognosis
- Apraxia
- Perseveration phenomena
- Hyperorality
- Insatiable appetite without weight gain
- Alexia
- Auditory agnosia
- Socially acceptable behaviors forgotten
- Hypertonia
- Unsteady gait

*From Hogstel, MO: *Clinical manual of gerontological nursing*, St. Louis, 1992, Mosby Year-Book, Inc.

- Agraphia

Symptoms of Stage Three
- Marked irritability
- Paraphasia
- Seizures
- Hyperorality
- Loss or diminution of emotions
- Bulimia
- Visual agnosia
- Hypermetamorphosis
- Apraxia
- Decreased appetite
- Bedridden
- Emaciated
- Helpless

Interventions

Since it is not possible to cure or arrest the progression of Alzheimer's disease, treatment is directed toward providing safety, meeting self-care needs, and meeting nutritional requirements. Pharmacologic agents such as haloperidol (Haldol), thiothixene (Navane), loxapine (Loxitane), and thioridazine (Mellaril) are prescribed to control the behavioral aspects of the disorder (Bauvette-Risey, 1989). Caregivers need factual information regarding the progression of Alzheimer's disease, as well as assistance in locating community support groups. Families may also need information and counsel in determining the appropriateness of institutional care.

The prognosis is poor. The disease often lasts from 5 to 20 years, and the physical, psychological, and financial problems encountered by the caregivers are immeasurable.

Alzheimer Client/
Family Education: Client Safety*

- Have client wear an identification band with name, address, and phone number.
- Install an alarm system or special locks on doors.
- Secure car keys.
- Ensure that client is always appropriately dressed for weather (in case of wandering).
- Place all medications in a locked medicine cabinet.
- Place all cleaning compounds/poisons in a locked cabinet.
- Keep a bathroom or hallway light on at night.
- Keep environment free of unnecessary furniture, and do not rearrange living area.
- Bedroom should be on ground floor if at all possible. If bedroom is upstairs, install stair guard.

*From Hogstel, MO: *Clinical manual of gerontological nursing*, St. Louis, 1992, Mosby Year-Book, Inc.

Pain Management

A large number of home care clients experience pain. As early discharge results in sicker clients seen in the home, the number needing assistance with pain control is increasing. Also, pain management is a central component of hospice care. It is therefore important to assess all clients for the presence of pain.

Misconceptions About the Pain Experience

Nurses often hear that it is crucial both to ask clients about their pain experiences and to believe their responses, but actual practices do not reflect this. In reality, clients frequently do not receive effective pain management because of some commonly held misbeliefs that are used as a basis for practice. These erroneous beliefs make solutions to pain management more difficult than is necessary. Table 25 summarizes some common misconceptions about pain.

Table 25   Misconceptions About Assessment of Clients Who Indicate They Have Pain

Misconception	Correction
The health team is the authority about the existence and nature of the client's pain sensation.	The person with pain is the only authority about the existence and nature of that pain, since the sensation of pain can be felt only by the person who has it.
Our personal values and intuition about the trustworthiness of others is a valuable tool in identifying whether a person is lying about pain.	Personal values and intuition do not constitute a professional approach to the client with pain. The client's credibility is not on trial.

(Continued)

Table 25 Misconceptions About Assessment of Clients Who Indicate They Have Pain (cont'd)

Misconception	Correction
Pain is largely an emotional or psychological problem, especially in the client who is highly anxious or depressed.	Having an emotional reaction to pain does not mean that pain is caused by an emotional problem. If anxiety or depression is alleviated, the intensity of pain will not necessarily be any less.
Lying about the existence of pain, malingering, is common.	Very few people who say they have pain are lying about it. Outright fabrication of pain is considered rare.
The client who obtains benefits or preferential treatment because of pain is receiving secondary gain and does not hurt as much as he says or may not hurt at all.	The client who uses his pain to his advantage is not the same as a malingerer and may still hurt as much as he says he does. Also, secondary gain may be an inaccurate diagnosis.
All real pain has an identifiable physical cause.	All pain is real, regardless of its cause. Almost all pain has both physical and mental components. Pure psychogenic pain is rare.
Visible signs, either physiological or behavioral, accompany pain and can be used to verify its existence and severity.	Even with severe pain, periods of physiological and behavioral adaptation occur, leading to periods of minimal or no signs of pain. Lack of pain expression does not necessarily mean lack of

(Continued)

Table 25   Misconceptions About Assessment of Clients Who Indicate They Have Pain (cont'd)

Misconception	Correction
	pain. How must the client act for us to believe she has pain?
Comparable physical stimuli produce comparable pain in different people. The severity and duration of pain can be predicted accurately for everyone on the basis of the stimuli for pain.	Comparable stimuli in different people do not produce the same intensities of pain. Comparable stimuli in different people will produce different intensities of pain that last different periods. There is no direct and invariant relationship between any stimulus and the perception of pain.
People with pain should be taught to have a high tolerance for pain. The more prolonged the pain or the more experience a person has with pain, the better is her tolerance for pain.	Pain tolerance is the individual's unique response, varying between clients and varying in the same client from one situation to another. People with prolonged pain tend to have an increasingly low pain tolerance. Respect for the client's pain tolerance is crucial for adequate pain control.
When the client reports pain relief following a placebo, this means that the client is a malingerer or that the pain is psychogenic.	There is not a shred of evidence anywhere in the literature to justify using a placebo to diagnose malingering or psychogenic pain.

McCaffery M and Beebe A: *Pain: Clinical manual for nursing practice*, St. Louis, 1989, The C.V. Mosby Company.

Misconceptions About Pain in the Elderly*

MYTH: Pain is expected with aging.

FACT: Pain is not normal with aging. The presence of pain in the elderly necessitates aggressive assessment, diagnosis, and management similar to that of younger clients.

MYTH: Pain sensitivity and perception decrease with aging.

FACT: This assumption is dangerous! Data are conflicting regarding age-associated changes in pain perception, sensitivity, and tolerance. Consequences of this assumption are needless suffering and undertreatment of both pain and the underlying cause.

MYTH: If a client does not complain of pain, he or she must not have much pain.

FACT: This is erroneous in all ages but particularly in the elderly. Older clients may not report pain for a variety of reasons. They may fear the meaning of the pain, diagnostic workups, or pain treatments. They may think pain is normal.

MYTH: A person who has no functional impairment, appears occupied, or is otherwise distracted from pain must not have significant pain.

FACT: Clients have a variety of reactions to pain. Many clients are stoic and refuse to "give in" to their pain. Over extended periods of time, the elderly may mask any outward signs of pain.

MYTH: Narcotic medications are inappropriate for clients with chronic nonmalignant pain.

FACT: Opioid analgesics are often indicated in nonmalignant pain.

MYTH: Potential side effects of narcotic medications make them too dangerous to use in the elderly.

FACT: Narcotics may be used safely in the elderly. Although elderly clients may be more sensitive to narcotics, this does not justify withholding narcotics and failing to relieve pain.

*Watt-Watson JH and Donavan MI: *Pain management: A nursing perspective*, St. Louis, 1992, Mosby-Year Book, Inc.

Pain is often not managed well at home. This is due to many factors such as family fears about drug addiction and tolerance, inadequate knowledge about basic pain management principles, and the fear that they might administer a lethal dose of medication. Also, in some cases, caregivers may deny that a client is experiencing pain to avoid confronting the reality that the client's condition has worsened (Creasia, 1991).

Assessment of Pain

In home health care, the nurse has the key role in assessing the adequacy of pain management and advocating for successful pain management. A brief assessment incorporates (LaRocca, 1994):

- The client's pain rating
- Description of the pain
- Onset, location, and duration of pain
- Any associated activity
- Medications used for pain relief
- Any behavioral component

A long-term assessment will involve client education and client choice in selecting the alternatives available for pain management. Past experience with pain, cultural factors, religion, and anxiety also need to be considered as they relate to the current experience. The home health nurse needs to monitor pain level, integrity of access devices, mental status, bowel function, and side effects from narcotics used, on each visit for possible adjustment.

On each visit the nurse should evaluate the following:

- Complications of the devices used to deliver the analgesic, which may range from connector problems to errors of pump programming
- Degree of pain experienced, including location, intensity, and quality
- Mental status
- Effectiveness of established bowel regimen
- All medications used by the client, including over-the-counter medications, street drugs, and alcohol
- Presence of side effects that are troublesome to the client, including nausea, orthostatic hypotension, urinary retention, and pruritis
- Caregiver and client feelings and coping

The following tools may be used to assess a client's pain. At the same time, since treatment of underlying conditions is the most important aspect of pain management, an accurate diagnosis is essential.

Initial Pain Assessment Tool

Date
Client's Name   Age
Diagnosis   Physician
                               Nurse

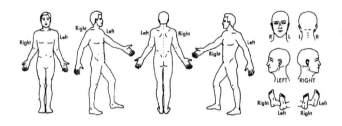

   I. Location: Client or nurse mark drawing.
   II. Intensity: Client rates the pain. Scale used.

Present:
Worst pain gets:
Best pain gets:
Acceptable level of pain:

   III. Quality: (Use client's own words, e.g., prick, ache, burn, throb, pull, sharp.)

   IV. Onset, Duration Variations, Rhythms:

   V. Manner of Expressing Pain:

   VI. What Relieves the Pain?

   VII. What Causes or Increases the Pain?

(Continued)

Initial Pain Assessment Tool (cont'd)

VIII. Effects of Pain: (Note decreased function,
      decreased quality of life.)
Accompanying symptoms (e.g., nausea)
Sleep
Appetite
Physical activity
Relationship with others (e.g., irritability)
Emotions (e.g., anger, suicidal, crying)
Concentration
Other

IX. Other Comments:

X. Plan:

From McCaffery M and Beebe A: *Pain: Clinical manual for nursing practice*, St. Louis, 1989, The C.V. Mosby Company.

Pain Questionnaire

1. Are you having pain right now? Yes___ No___ Please mark an X at the spot that best describes your pain right now.

NO   _____ WORST
PAIN   POSSIBLE
                                              PAIN

2. If you are pain free now, when did you last have pain?

3. About how often have you had pain this week?

4. In general, was your pain this week:
   ___Constant   ___ Periodic   ___ Brief
   (never free of pain) (comes and goes) (less than 15 min.)

(Continued)

Pain Questionnaire (cont'd)

5. Please mark an X at the spot that describes the *least* pain you had this week.

NO   _____   WORST
PAIN   POSSIBLE
                                            PAIN

6. Please mark an X at the spot that describes the *worst* pain you had this week.

NO   _____   WORST
PAIN   POSSIBLE
                                            PAIN

7. Overall how would you rate your pain this week?
   - 0   no pain
   - 1   mild
   - 2   discomforting
   - 3   distressing
   - 4   horrible
   - 5   excruciating

Watt-Watson JH and Donavan MI: *Pain management: A nursing perspective*, St. Louis, 1992, Mosby-Year Book, Inc.

Pharmacologic Management of Pain

Most clients identified for home pain management have intractable pain and require a narcotic infusion along with adjuvant therapy. There are three groups of analgesics used to manage pain: nonnarcotics, narcotics (opioids), and adjuvant medications.

Nonnarcotics

Nonnarcotics act on the peripheral nervous system. Acetaminophen, aspirin, and nonsteroidal antiinflammatory drugs (NSAIDs) are included in this group. Most nonnarcotic drugs are powerful antiinflammatories and inhibit the synthesis of prostaglandin.

Table 26   Nonnarcotic Pain Relieving Agents

Generic Name	Trade Name	Usual Oral Daily Dosages
Acetylated Salicylates		
Acetylsalicylic acid (ASA)	Aspirin	650-1000 mg QID
Nonacetylated Salicylates		
Choline magnesium trisalicylate	Trilisate	1500 mg BID
Diflunisal	Dolobid	500-1000 mg BID
Salsalate	Disalcid*	750 mg QID
Para-aminophenol Derivatives		
Acetaminophen	Tylenol	650-1000 mg QID
Proprionic Acid Derivatives		
Fenoprofen	Nalfon	200-600 mg TID or QID
Flurbiprofen	Ansaid	150-300 mg TID or QID
Ibuprofen	Advil, Motrin, Nuprin, Rufen	400-800 mg TID or QID
Ketoprofen	Orudis	50-75 mg TID or QID
Naproxen	Naprosyn	250-500 mg BID
Naproxen sodium	Anaprox	275 mg TID or QID
Tiaprofenic acid	Surgam	600 mg BID or TID
Indole Acetic Acid Derivatives		
Indomethacin	Indocin, Indocid	25-50 mg BID or TID
Sulindac	Clinoril	150-200 mg BID

(Continued)

Table 26 Nonnarcotic Pain Relieving Agents (cont'd)

Generic Name	Trade Name	Usual Oral Daily Dosages
Oxicams		
Piroxicam	Feldene	20 mg QID
Pyrazolones		
Phenylbutazone	Butazolidin	100-200 mg TID
Oxyphenbutazone	Tandearil	100 mg TID or QID
Sulfinpyrazone	Anturan, 200-800 mg BID Anturane	
Anthranilic Acids		
Meclofenamate	Meclomen	200-400 mg TID or QID
Mefenamic acid	Ponstan	250 mg TID
Floctafenine	Idarac	200-400 mg TID or QID
Pyrrole-acetic Acid		
Tolmetin sodium	Tolectin	400-600 mg BID or TID
Ketorolac tromethamine	Toradol	15-30 mg IM QID (not available in oral formuations)
Phenylacetic Acid		
Diclofenac sodium	Voltaren	100-150 mg BID or TID

*United States only.

Watt-Watson JH and Donavan MI: *Pain management: A nursing perspective,* St. Louis, 1992, Mosby-Year Book, Inc.

Narcotics

Narcotics—primarily the opiates—work centrally when given through various routes such as oral, sublingual, rectal, transdermal, intramuscular, and subcutaneous. Narcotics are classified as weak narcotics, to be used for mild to moderate pain, and strong narcotics.

Table 27   Opiates

Generic Name / Trade Name	Equianalgesic Dosages (mg)		Duration of Action (hr)
	IM	PO	
Weak Agonists			
Codeine /	130	200	3-4
Tylenol #1 = 7.5 mg with 300 mg acetaminophen			
Tylenol #2 = 15 mg with 300 mg acetaminophen			
Tylenol #3 = 30 mg with 300 mg acetaminophen			
Tylenol #4 = 60 mg with 300 mg acetaminophen			
Empirin #2 = 15 mg with 325 mg aspirin			
Empirin #3 = 30 mg with 325 mg aspirin			
Empirin #4 = 60 mg with 325 mg aspirin			
Propoxyphene /	—	500	3-4
Darvon			
Darvocet-N 50 = 50 mg with 325 mg acetaminophen			
Darvocet-N 100 = 100 mg with 650 mg acetaminophen			
Darvon-N with ASA = 100 mg with 325 mg aspirin			
Hydrocodone /	—	100	3-4
Lortab = 5 mg with 500 mg acetaminophen			
Lortab 7.5 = 7.5 mg with 500 mg acetaminophen			
Vicodin = 5 mg with 500 mg acetaminophen			
Vicodin ES = 7.5 mg with 500 acetaminophen			
Oxycodone /	—	30	3-4
Roxicodone*			

(Continued)

Table 27 Opiates (cont'd)

Generic Name / Trade Name	Equianalgesic Dosages (mg)		Duration of Action (hr)
	IM	PO	

Percodan = 5 mg oxycodone and 325 mg aspirin
Percocet = 5 mg oxycodone and 325 mg acetaminophen
Tylox* = 5 mg oxycodone and 500 mg acetaminophen

Generic Name / Trade Name	IM	PO	Duration (hr)
Strong Agonists			
Morphine	10	60 (20-30)	4
sustained release			8-12
Fentanyl / Sublimaze	0.05 (IV)	—	1 1/2
Hydromorphone / Dilaudid	1.5	7.5	2-4
Levorphanol / Levo-Dromoran	2	4	4
Meperidine / Demerol	75	300	3-4 IM 12-16 oral
Methadone / Dolophine	10	20	3-5 (may be as long as 12-24 hours)
Oxymorphone / Numorphan	1	—	3-4
rectal	10		4-6
Partial Agonist			
Buprenorphine* / Buprenex	0.4	—	6

(Continued)

Table 27   Opiates (cont'd)

Generic Name / Trade Name	Equianalgesic Dosages (mg)		Duration of Action (hr)
	IM	PO	
Mixed Agonists-Antagonists			
Dezocine / Dalgan	10	—	3-4
Butorphanol / Stadol	2	—	3-4
Nalbuphine / Nubain	10	—	3-6
Pentazocine / Talwin	60	180	3

*United States only.

Watt-Watson JH and Donavan MI: *Pain management: A nursing perspective,* St. Louis, 1992, Mosby-Year Book, Inc.

New Methods of Opiate Delivery

Research has focused on providing new methods of delivering opiates. Many of these new methods are creative alternatives that circumvent potential obstacles that occur with previously used techniques. These include methods to deliver drugs when clients cannot take opiates orally and strategies that circumvent side effects associated with traditional routes. The following table highlights the advantages and disadvantages of each route (Watt-Watson, 1992).

Table 28 Opiate Delivery Routes

Route	Advantages	Disadvantages
Oral	Ease of administration, reduced morbidity (absence of injection pain or hematomas and risk of cellulitis). Reduced cost (does not require purchase of syringes or needles).	Duration of action of most opiates is approximately 4 hours; clients with chronic pain have been forced to awaken several times during the night to medicate themselves for pain.
Sustained release morphine tablets (MS Contin, Roxane)	Allows gradual breakdown of the drug; clients receive continuous relief over 8 to 12 hours.	
High concentration liquid morphine	Allows clients who can swallow only small amounts to continue taking the drug by mouth.	
Transdermal	Alternative therapy for persons who cannot take oral medications. Relatively stable plasma drug level; noninvasive. Each patch provides delivery of drug for 72 hours.	Systemic side effects: nausea and vomiting and somnolence. Local reactions to the patch include erythema and rash. Specific questions that remain unanswered are the effects of hydration on absorption, as well as the influence of cachexia and reduced fat stores on drug availability.

(Continued)

Table 28   Opiate Delivery Routes (cont'd)

Route	Advantages	Disadvantages
Intravenous	More rapid onset of action and stable blood levels when delivered continuously; precludes the need for painful injections. Provides relief with few side effects. Established safety. Intravenous morphine can be delivered over extended time with relative ease via ambulatory infusion pumps.	
Sublingual/Buccal	Benefits those who cannot swallow or who have a bowel obstruction.	Taste is not palatable. Clients should be discouraged from swallowing the drug and should not eat or drink within 15 minutes of applying the drug.
Rectal	Useful for clients who have dysphagia or nausea and vomiting. Rectal suppositories are also convenient to administer.	

(Continued)

Table 28 Opiate Delivery Routes (cont'd)

Route	Advantages	Disadvantages
Subcutaneous catheters and infusion pumps	Clients without permanent venous access devices can receive continuous infusions of drug in the home setting. Small-gauged catheters allow ease of administration.	Poor absorption is usually due to fibrosis at insertion site and is evidenced by a decrease in analgesic effect. High concentrations of opiate delivery are necessary to allow delivery of adequate dose in a small volume of fluid.
Intraspinal (epidural or intrathecal) infusion	Reduction of side effects seen with systemic opiates due to direct action of the drug on opiate receptors in the dorsal horn of the spinal cord. Few side effects, if any, occur.	Sedation, constipation, nausea, and vomiting, due to binding of the drug to opiate receptors throughout the brain and GI tract. Risk of infection with external catheters. Higher opiate dose needed with epidural route.

Adapted from Watt-Watson JH and Donavan MI: *Pain management: A nursing perspective*, St. Louis, 1992, Mosby-Year Book, Inc.

Combining Opiates and NSAIDs

Because NSAIDs and opiates have different mechanisms of action, it is often useful to combine these agents. In fact, commercially available formulations that include both categories (e.g., codeine and acetaminophen) capitalize on these different mechanisms, providing analgesia while causing fewer side effects than if a higher dose of one drug were used.

The World Health Organization recommends a sequential, or three-step ladder, approach to the management of cancer pain. This approach, or modifications of this approach, might be applicable to types of pain other than cancer. Initial therapy begins with an NSAID (Step 1). When the client receives the maximum recommended dose of NSAIDs and continues to experience pain, one adds a weak opiate (Step 2). The dose of the weak opiate is increased until relief is obtained, side effects occur, or the ceiling dose is reached. If an adequate dose of a weak opiate does not provide relief, one changes to a stronger opiate (Step 3). At any time during therapy, an adjuvant drug may be added (Watt-Watson, 1992).

Adjuvant Drugs

Adjuvant drugs are defined as drugs that are primarily used for conditions other than pain relief. These drugs include anticonvulsants, antidepressants, neuroleptics, anxiolytics, and corticosteroids. It is important to note that these drugs do not replace NSAIDs or opiates but merely serve to augment the pain relief associated with analgesics or to act as options for relief when adequate doses of analgesics fail (Watt-Watson, 1992).

Maintaining Blood Levels of Analgesics

To achieve effective pain relief in severe pain, analgesics must be given around the clock to maintain blood levels of the drugs. Peaks and troughs of analgesia are eliminated by around-the-clock administration, and pain-associated anxiety is decreased or eliminated.

An around-the-clock (ATC) schedule, rather than prn administration, is most appropriate when clients have pain that lingers during the day (American Pain Society, 1989). The interval between doses is based on the duration of action of the drug being delivered. A drug with a duration of action of 4 hours should be given at least every 4 hours to preclude a reduction in therapeutic blood levels. Administering the next dose of drug only when the person is in pain (the prn approach) ensures the need for higher doses of analgesics and far more time for drug absorption. In pain of longer duration, a combination of ATC dosing for baseline pain and prn dosing for intermittent increasing pain (breakthrough pain) may be necessary (Portenoy, 1989).

Requesting a Change of Analgesic Orders From a Physician

Before notifying the physician, be certain the current analgesics have:

- Been given at the prescribed interval
- Been given around the clock, with no doses omitted
- Remained in the body long enough to be effective (i.e., vomiting and diarrhea have not appeared)
- Been given for an appropriate number of days
- Been documented as ineffective using a flow sheet

Communication About Ineffective Analgesia

Documentation should include (Watt-Watson, 1992):

- Client's name
- Period of time drug has been tried
- Current drug(s) amount, frequency of administration, and last change in dosage
- Rating scale being used
- 24-hour average pain rating, including highest and lowest rating
- (If narcotics) Respiratory rate, level of awareness, and whether the client can sleep/rest
- Drug side effects client is currently experiencing on this dosage
- Nondrug measures currently being used for pain relief
- Request for suggestions from physician for more effective use of current drugs; if the physician has no suggestions, be prepared to *suggest* alternative

Client/Family Teaching Point:
Your Concerns About Addiction

To: _____ Date:_____
                Client's name

The fears you or your family may have about addiction could:
- Prevent you from requesting or taking the pain medication
- Result in your holding off as long as possible between doses
- Result in your taking lower doses of medication even though pain is not controlled

Doing any of the above will only result in needless suffering. Talk to the nurses about your concerns and fears. They will help you learn the facts about addiction:
1. Addiction very rarely happens in people who are taking pain medication to relieve pain.
2. Being on narcotics a long time does not increase your chance of becoming addicted.
3. When the pain stops or is less, most people are able to stop or reduce their pain medication without any problem.

Ask yourself "Is there any reason that I would want to take this narcotic when I no longer have pain?" If you can answer no, then you will be able to stop taking the medication when the pain stops.

Additional comments:

If you have any questions or concerns about the above, contact:

_____   _____
       RN or MD name   Phone

_____
       Nurse's signature

From McCaffery M and Beebe A: *Pain: Clinical manual for nursing practice,* St. Louis, 1989, The C.V. Mosby Company.

Table 29   Guidelines for Effective Use of Nonnarcotic Analgesics

Guideline	Comment
Weigh risk vs. benefits in selection.	e.g, aspirin: risk of GI upset but it is least expensive in this group; acetaminophen: less antiinflammatory effect but generally fewer side effects.
Start with a low dose to determine side effects, etc. Increase gradually to dose that relieves pain, not exceeding maximal daily dose.	May need to increase to 1-2 times the starting dose. Ineffective analgesia may be due to inadequate doses.
If maximal antiinflammatory effect is desired in addition to analgesia, allow adequate trial before discontinuing or switching.	An effective dose should provide pain relief within 2 hours. Maximal anti-inflammatory effect occurs later as drug accumulates. With regular doses for 1 week or longer, pain relief may increase.
If one drug becomes ineffective, but the pain is about the same, try a drug from a different chemical class (see table on NSAIDs).	The inflammatory process may have changed. A different drug may attack this process in another way.
If they do not relieve pain when used alone, combine with PO, IM, or IV narcotics for added analgesic effect.	Rationale: nonnarcotic analgesics stop pain at peripheral nervous system (PNS) level and narcotics stop pain at CNS level. Combination of PNS plus CNS attack will provide added analgesic effect.

From McCaffery M and Beebe A: *Pain: Clinical manual for nursing practice,* St. Louis, 1989, The C.V. Mosby Company.

Nonpharmacological Pain Management

Pharmacological pain management *alone* is often not adequate. Also, pharmacological analgesics, particularly narcotics, are not appropriate for some clients. Several alternate therapies involve some form of peripheral or central stimulation to manage pain. Varying degrees of success have been reported.

Nurses have traditionally focused on the whole person and family. Because nonpharmacological pain management techniques often involve a holistic approach, the nurse is uniquely prepared for effective use of these techniques.

The following sections provide an overview of the various nonpharmacological, research-based options that are available to nurses for the management of pain along with guidelines for their use. All techniques meet the following criteria:

- The average nurse is qualified to use them effectively, although some special training may be necessary.
- They do not require special equipment that is not readily available.
- They do not interfere with any medical treatments the client may be undergoing.
- They do not require the client's official informed consent.

Health professionals will undoubtedly continue to use pharmacological methods as the principal form of pain treatment. However, in selected clients, nonpharmacological techniques used alone or in combination with pain medications often provide a significant and improved form of pain relief (Watt-Watson, 1992).

Peripheral Techniques

Peripheral techniques are those interventions involving stimulation of the skin to reduce pain. They can be used to treat a wide variety of acute and chronic pains. In this section the following interventions are discussed: cryotherapy, superficial heat, massage, acupressure, and transcutaneous electrical nerve stimulation (TENS). As pain is a unique, subjective experience, the clinician must implement various measures in different combinations to design the optimum program for each individual (Watt-Watson, 1992).

Cryotherapy

Mechanisms of Action

Can reduce release of pain-causing chemicals such as lactic acid, potassium ions, kinins, serotonin, and histamine. Also decreases lymph production and cell permeability, resulting in diminished edema formation and subsequent pain reduction. Can slow conduction velocity of small unmyelinated nerve fibers, which conduct pain impulses from the periphery. When acupuncture points are massaged with cold (ice massage), afferent stimulation is thought to activate brain stem mechanisms that are known to exert descending inhibitory influences on pain signals. Afferent stimulation achieved with ice massage of an acupoint is thought to be of higher intensity than when other areas of the body surface are similarly treated. Therefore the analgesic effect is greater.

Clinical Uses and Contraindications

Particularly useful for initial post-traumatic pain, swelling, and muscle spasm. Also recommended for relief of pain associated with chronic ischemic ulcers. Ice massage has reportedly been helpful for a variety of pain types including musculoskeletal, myofascial, and acute dental pain. Contraindicated for clients with peripheral vascular disease with arterial insufficiency, Raynaud's phenomenon, cold allergy, paroxysmal cold hemoglobinuria, marked cold pressure response, or any indication of cold sensitivity. Also contraindicated for clients with heart disease and angina pectoris.

Guidelines for Use

Many methods of cold therapy are available. Usually some type of cold pack or ice pack (wooden spatula placed in a cupful of water, frozen, and covered with a moist towel) is applied to the affected area. Limit contact time to 15 minutes per session to avoid frostbite. With ice massage, an ice pack is massaged over the involved acupoints or painful area for no longer than 7 minutes.

Nursing's Role

Cryotherapy is often an effective analgesic. This therapeutic modality is inexpensive, requires little nursing time, and can easily be taught to the client and/or the family. Therefore nurses have a responsibility to try this technique and, if successful, incorporate it into their client's pain treatment program.

Superficial Heat

Mechanisms of Action

Application of moist or dry heat to the body's surface. Indirectly, once an inflammatory response has subsided, heat can reduce pain through a vasodilator effect. Vasodilation enhances blood flow, causing improvements in tissue nutrition and elimination of cellular metabolites that stimulate pain impulses. Heat triggers pain-inhibiting reflexes through temperature receptors. Both of these actions result in relaxation of muscle spasm and an associated reduction in pain. Elevation of surface body temperature can also cause reactions distant from the site of temperature elevation. For example, superficial heat has been observed to relax smooth musculature of the gastrointestinal tract, which in turn reduces the pain of gastrointestinal cramps.

Superficial heat also has direct influence on pain. Evidence suggests that the application of heat to a peripheral nerve or the skin increases the pain threshold in that area, although not as effectively as cryotherapy. However, studies have shown that clients do prefer heat to cold.

Clinical Uses and Contraindications

Especially effective for muscle and joint pain, but contraindicated after trauma and on tissues with inadequate circulation. Heating of tissues with inadequate circulation increases metabolic demands while tissue oxygenation remains inadequate. The combination of these reactions can lead to ischemic necrosis. Do not apply heat to a malignancy site unless client is terminal. Use with caution over areas with impaired sensation or in clients with limited or no ability to communicate.

Guidelines for Use

Commonly applied with hot water bottles, electric heating pads, moist towels, warm baths, infrared apparatus, or the summer sun. Treatment should be limited to 1/2 hour 3 to 4 times per day to avoid thermal injury.

Nursing's Role

Like cryotherapy, heat is an effective analgesic and is inexpensive, simple to use, and not time consuming. Therefore, in appropriate cases, nurses should assess the effectiveness of this modality and incorporate it into the pain-treatment plan if it proves successful.

Massage

Mechanisms of Action

Little is known about the mechanism by which massage produces analgesia. The mechanical pressure of massage on superficial venous and lymphatic channels improves circulation directly, reducing the pain associated with edema. Second, massage causes capillary and, if strong enough, arteriole dilation through some unknown reflex mechanism. This further improves circulation.

More recently Day, Mason, and Chesrown (1987) evaluated the effect of massage on plasma beta-endorphin levels in 21 healthy adults before and after a 30-minute back massage. They found no significant differences in plasma beta-endorphin levels but recommended a similar study be carried out on those suffering acute or chronic pain. In 1989, Kaada and Torsteinbo carried out such a study on 12 volunteers suffering from myalgia and various other types of pain. They noted a 16% significant increase in plasma beta-endorphins after 30 minutes of connective tissue massage, suggesting that the analgesic action of massage may be mediated, at least in part, by the release of endorphins.

Clinical Uses and Contraindications

Anecdotal reports suggest that massage is applicable for most client populations. Contraindications have not been fully delineated. Obvious indications for avoiding massage in the area of concern include conditions involving fractures, phlebitis, skin lesions, lacerations, and recent surgery or injury.

Guidelines for Use

As a therapeutic intervention, massage consists of five basic movements or strokes used in sequence on the body's surface: effleurage, petrissage, friction, tapotement, and vibration.

Nursing's Role

Inexpensive, reasonably easy-to-learn technique but requires much time to perform. However, because of its simplicity, family members can carry out the treatment with relatively little instruction. At present, objective evidence of the therapeutic value of massage is scarce. Experimental studies now are needed concerning optimum forms, the best candidates, and the contraindications.

Acupressure

Mechanisms of Action

Technique involves applying finger pressure to points that correspond to many of the points used in acupuncture. Little is known of how acupressure exerts its analgesic effect. Both the acupoint and its immediate surrounding are richly endowed with nerves and pressure and stretch receptors. Further, they are points of decreased electrical resistance, suggesting that these areas are particularly susceptible to pressure and/or electrical stimulation. It has been hypothesized that acupressure stimulates pressure fibers, which belong to the larger, myelinated, and rapidly conducting category of afferents. When stimulated, the pressure fibers function to "close" the gating mechanism in the spinal cord to impulses from the small unmyelinated and slower conducting nerve fibers that transmit pain impulses from the periphery. Also, there is some evidence suggesting endorphins are released when specific acupoints are pressed.

Clinical Uses and Contraindications

Many pain complaints have been treated with acupressure. Good results are reported when combined with progressive relaxation techniques. Contraindicated in pregnant women, because several acupoints are believed to have powerful oxytocic effects.

Guidelines for Use

The location and probable etiology of the client's pain will determine which acupoints should be treated. A variety of acupressure techniques are taught in the West. Generally, the basic technique is as follows:

1. *Locate the specific acupoint.* Because acupoints exhibit a lower electrical resistance than the immediate surrounding areas, they can be located with commercially available electrical point locators. However, it is reported that acupoints can be identified by touch. The acupoints are said to feel softer and more yielding than the adjacent skin surfaces, and finger pressure can elicit tenderness and/or pain.

2. *Stimulate the acupoint.* Pressure can be applied with either a finger, thumb, or knuckle. Preferably, pressure is increased

to the client's level of tolerance. Reference sources include Weaver, Penzer and Matsumoto, and Beggs. Most therapists practice rotating the finger either slowly or briskly in a circular or spiral motion for anywhere from 15 seconds to 5 minutes.

3. *Check for effectiveness.* After the treatment, assess the degree of relief and client satisfaction. If the effect was not fully satisfactory, another point should be stimulated. In cases of extreme tenderness at the primary point, treating the same point on the contralateral side may be helpful.

Nursing's Role

Acupressure is a simple, safe, inexpensive, and noninvasive technique that requires little time to learn or perform. As such, nurses familiar with the technique can use it in an attempt to reduce or alleviate pain. In addition, if the treatment proves effective, they can teach the specific technique to the client in pain and/or his or her relatives.

Transcutaneous Electrical Nerve Stimulation (TENS)

Mechanisms of Action

The gate control theory has generated a variety of methods to control pain, including TENS. Basically this treatment involves passing a mild electric current across the skin between two electrodes. By altering the stimulation parameters, several different types of TENS can be produced. Evidence suggests that the various types of TENS exert their analgesic effect by one or a combination of two mechanisms. The first involves activating large-diameter, myelinated A beta fibers, closing the gate to pain impulses from the periphery. The second mechanism appears to involve deep fiber activation, followed by endorphin release in some cases.

Clinical Uses and Contraindications

Clinicians and researchers have used TENS to treat a wide variety of both acute and chronic pain types. Collectively the findings suggest that TENS is an effective modality for some but not all pain types. Contraindications are few. TENS is not recommended for those with contact dermatitis or in early pregnancy and should be used only with careful evaluation and extended cardiac monitoring for those with cardiac pacemakers.

Guidelines for Use

A physician's prescription is usually required. Unwanted side effects directly attributable to TENS are rare and relatively minor. The most common is contact dermatitis. This problem usually disappears when treatment is stopped, electrode gel changed, or electrode placement adjusted.

The TENS unit consists of two to four electrodes connected by lead wires to a stimulator. The TENS stimulus consists of three parameters, intensity, frequency, and pulse width, which can be adjusted on the stimulator to create the different types of TENS. The stimulus parameters of three of the more commonly used modes are shown in Table 30. Successful treatment depends on adequately varying the stimulus parameters and electrode placement until the best results are achieved. There are many options for electrode placement, including site of pain, acupuncture points, spinal nerve roots, and contralateral side.

Regardless of the type of pain being treated, TENS is rarely used alone but rather serves as an adjunct to other forms of pain management, such as medication. TENS does not require highly skilled and frequent nursing care to ensure effective use. TENS units are expensive to purchase but cost little to maintain, provided they are not lost, stolen, or damaged.

Nursing's Role

Many facilities employ either TENS technicians or physiotherapists who provide the client with the instrument and properly teach the client to use it. As part of the pain management team, the nurse can recommend the use of TENS for specific clients. Therefore they can reinforce the instruction provided to the client, assist the client in experimenting with different settings and electrode placement sites, and trouble shoot.

Table 30 Stimulus Parameters of the Three More Commonly Used Modes of TENS

Stimulus Parameters	TENS Mode		
	Conventional	Acupuncture-like	Intense
Intensity	To tolerable tingling sensation	To tolerable muscle contraction	Just below muscle contraction
Frequency (pulses/sec)	80-125	2-4 or a series of high frequency pulses delivered in bursts of 2-4/sec	125
Pulse width (microseconds)	60-100	220-250	250

Watt-Watson JH and Donavan MI: *Pain management: A nursing perspective,* St. Louis, 1992, Mosby-Year Book, Inc.

Central Techniques

Central techniques are thought to exert their effect through alteration of sensory, evaluative, and/or affective factors. They include relaxation, cognitive strategies, imagery, music, distraction, and positive suggestion (Watt-Watson, 1992).

Relaxation

Mechanisms of Action

Characterized by decreased oxygen consumption, muscle tonus, and heart and respiratory rate; lowered arterial blood lactate; increased skin resistance; intense, slow alpha waves; and occasional theta activity in the brain. The relaxation response may reduce distressing thoughts and feelings by reducing anxiety. As anxiety and relaxation produce opposite physiological results, clearly they cannot exist together. The most commonly used form of relaxation training is progressive muscle relaxation.

Clinical Uses and Precautions

Knowing the pattern and intensity of the client's pain is essential in deciding whether relaxation may be helpful. Clients with very mild pain may not be good candidates for relaxation training because they may not be motivated to expend the time and effort needed for learning. Clients with severe pain may require simpler or more other-directed techniques. Probably the best candidates are those with moderately severe acute or chronic pain that is not well controlled by analgesics or that is well controlled but with unwanted side effects and clients undergoing procedural pain.

Guidelines for Use

Relaxation techniques vary in method, but all have several characteristics in common:

1. A quiet environment
2. A comfortable position that enhances decreased muscle tonus
3. A passive, "let it happen" attitude and an ability to disregard distracting thoughts and redirect them toward the technique
4. A mental device such as a word, sound, or phrase that can help shift thoughts from an external to an internal orientation

Adequate client preparation is critical for the success of relaxation training. First, reassure clients that pain itself is a major contributor to stress, which in turn increases pain. Relaxation reduces pain in at least two ways—by diminishing the sensation of pain and by allowing the client to control the intensity of his or her reaction to the pain. Suggest that clients keep their eyes open if they are initially uncomfortable with the passive, "let it go" approach necessary for success. Remind clients that they maintain complete control over how much relaxation they allow themselves to experience. Clients are instructed not to fall asleep while they are learning relaxation. Every relaxation session ends with a slow, paced return to normal activities, to prevent any dizziness or orthostatic hypotension.

Clients need to practice at least 3 times a week until they are comfortable and familiar with the exercise. Clients in pain may use it 2 to 3 times daily.

Nursing's Role

Progressive muscle relaxation cannot be carried out by either the nurse or client without considerable instruction and time. What nursing can accomplish within a brief time is creating an awareness of the technique and encouraging an interest in learning more about it. Giving the client a list of a few centers that teach relaxation may be useful. Some of the shorter relaxation procedures, particularly deep breathing with focusing, involve only minutes at a time and no additional costs.

Cognitive Strategies

Mechanisms of Action

Cognitive strategies for pain control refer to techniques that influence pain through the use of one's thoughts or cognitions. Directly altering the thoughts and appraisals that surround painful events affects descending cortical impulses to the spinal cord, as proposed in the gate control theory of pain. One's perceived ability to successfully manage and tolerate pain leads to improved coping.

Clinical Uses and Precautions

Cognitive strategies usually are proposed in a three-phased approach to implementation.

Phase 1: Make clients become aware of their own thoughts about pain. Clients can record the facts, thoughts, and feelings they have about pain so that they may become clear about whether it is a fact that is causing the distress or a thought emanating from the fact. Feelings result from the thought, not the fact. Negative thoughts reduce tolerance to pain and make it much more difficult to handle.

Phase 2: The client begins to apply coping strategies and one or more new cognitive approaches to the pain experience. Substituting more realistic and rational statements in place of excessively negative thoughts permits the client to reframe his or her own experience in a less distressing way. With practice over time such positive self-statements become second nature and enhance feelings of personal control and self-efficacy.

Phase 3: The client needs to rehearse the cognitive strategies to become at ease and proficient with them.

Cognitive appraisal, according to Lazarus and Folkman, is the process by which an individual interprets information in terms of its significance for his or her well-being and evaluates its personal meaning. Thus an event is perceived as irrelevant, benign, challenging, or threatening (primary appraisal). Then the individual assesses how well he or she can deal with the event at hand (secondary appraisal).

Guidelines for Use

Whether the nurse's role is to suggest these strategies, to work directly with the client on them, or to simply "plant seeds" about contributing pain factors, the following guidelines may be useful:

1. The client is the most significant person in the process.
2. It is essential to develop a collaborative team approach with the client as captain. Client centeredness and team collaboration are important whenever one treats pain and when cognitive approaches are to be employed.
3. The client must always be in control of the process, since his or her feedback determines the next step. The client is central to the pain, the process, and the control.
4. Encourage the client to observe his or her own behavior and thought processes.
5. Help the client identify cues in the environment that will prompt him or her to talk to self differently.
6. If the client is reluctant to "buy" into these approaches, suggest that he or she is actually enduring two kinds of pain, physical and emotional. Whether or not the physical pain can be readily eliminated, the other pains can be minimized.

Nursing's Role

Although cognitive strategies look inherently simple, a considerable amount of time can be taken up in discussion about the role of thoughts in pain reduction. Further, this dialogue best occurs in blocks of time rather than in short periods of a few minutes each. Some of this discussion can certainly take place while the nurse is occupied with physical tasks or procedures.

Imagery

Mechanisms of Action

Imagery is a mental representation of reality or fantasy and may use all five senses in its creation. The term *guided imagery* has been coined to reflect the purposeful development of an image or images for a specific goal—usually related to improving one's physiological processes, (pain, autonomic reactivity), mental state, self-image, performance, or behavior. Guided imagery is generally preceded by some form of relaxation, which is thought to facilitate image development.

Individuals have been shown to be able to control heart rate, skin temperature, blood pressure, and muscle tension through the process of biofeedback. When subjects were asked how they were able to bring about such physiological changes, they replied that they did so by imagining relaxing scenes and allowing themselves to relax. Reduced nausea, vomiting, and distress have been reported in cancer clients after chemotherapy when the subjects practiced guided imagery and relaxation. The link between pain management and guided imagery may be a function of an intermediary relaxation response and sense of well-being generated by the performance of guided imagery.

There are several reasons why guided imagery helps people deal with pain successfully. One explanation is that the distraction that results from focusing on a pleasant relaxing image adds to its effectiveness. Another is that clients who use guided imagery regain a sense of personal control and self-control, especially when they are encouraged and directed to create their own pleasant images. The relaxation that precedes and/or accompanies imagery also contributes to reduced muscle tension, anxiety, and pain.

Clinical Uses and Precautions

Perhaps the key function of guided imagery lies in its ability to alter how clients perceive the sensations of pain. Studies suggest that guided imagery produces longer tolerance and less self-reported pain than training in relaxation, although it has been suggested that relaxation and imagery strategies combine additively. The benefit of psychological approaches to pain management lies in reducing the fear and depression associated with pain, rather than the pain itself.

Guided imagery varies in whether it is self-guided or other-guided. Other-guided imagery occurs when the nurse guides the imagery development explicitly by leading the client through a prepared description of the scene to be imagined; self-guided imagery clients are instructed to use their own imagination to remember or create pleasant images. Guided imagery can be a particularly helpful strategy in conjunction with other pain management approaches for use in a wide range of acute and chronic pain states.

Guidelines for Use

There is no one right way to teach guided imagery or any other cognitive-behavioral intervention. Each nurse must learn and practice a technique so that he or she feels comfortable with it before employing it with clients. The nurse and the client become partners in a collaborative relationship in selecting the imagery that the client will develop and when and how he or she will use it.

Both the nurse and the client need to be aware that guided imagery is a skill that needs to be learned and practiced at times when the client is pain-free or nearly so.

There are two distinctly different approaches that imagery may take. One is in the direction away from the painful experience. This approach actually develops an "incompatible" image. It changes the situation into one in which pain is not present, allowing the client to feel once more in charge of his or her feelings. This method is most frequently used by nurses and other health care professionals. A common example involves imagining a pleasant out-of-doors scene, such as a meadow, lake, or forest. Another approach imagery can take is described as transformational, because it is directed toward the pain. Specific strategies that clients have reported to be helpful are:

1. Converting the pain to nonpain, e.g., turning the painful area into ice, rushing water, trickles of sand, or pressure caused by imaginary animals sitting on the area.
2. Imagining the pain to be a color and then converting it to another color, switching from a warm to a cool color or vice versa.
3. Determining the pain level on a 0 to 10 horizontal scale, and then slowly moving the indicator lever to a slightly lower number, while breathing slowly and deeply with each incremental decrease in the pain rating.

Nursing's Role

Imagery is inexpensive and requires only small amounts of time. The effective use of imagery requires that the nurse have an open mind and a responsiveness to the client's selection of images and how they can be adapted.

Music

Mechanisms of Action

Definitive explanations for the efficacy of music therapy are not currently known. It has been postulated that there may be a conditioned relaxation response or distraction effect because of enjoyable past associations. Another possible mechanism of action is that auditory stimuli may directly suppress pain neurologically.

Music can also encourage distraction or dissociation from unpleasant or painful stimuli through the development of imagery, increase the production of endorphins, and serve as a cue for relaxation.

Clinical Uses and Precautions

Helpful for obstetric clients, chronic pain clients, and postoperative and hospitalized cancer clients. Music therapy, like other nonpharmacological methods of pain control, is not meant to be used alone, nor is it meant to be used when pain is already at a peak intensity. Not all clients in pain wish to listen to music during or before painful episodes, and some find that they either cannot or do not wish to focus on the music. When one discusses the use of music with clients, it is important to ascertain their experience with music, their skills or interest in different types of music, and their current listening abilities. Instrumental selections are recommended over vocal selections.

Guidelines for Use

Although music is an easy-to-use modality, it is not enough to simply present the music to the client and instruct the client to listen to it. A clear set of instructions is required so that the client will become an active participant in his or her own care. The following guidelines from McCaffery & Beebe (1989) are particularly helpful:

1. Listen only to the music.
2. Feel the music lifting you upward.
3. Let each measure rhythmically flow through your body and relax the muscles.
4. Let yourself float through the air with the melody.

It is best to introduce the client to music therapy before pain becomes intense or before commencing a painful procedure, such as wound packing.

By encouraging the client to become involved in the process of active listening, the nurse activates several other cognitive and mental strategies. The client may conduct his or her own inner dialogue, which can focus attention on more pleasant and relaxing images. Both the nurse and the client can measure the effectiveness of music as a treatment modality for pain control by rating the level of distress caused by the pain on a 0-to-10 visual analogue or numerical scale before and after the listening session. Clients can then be encouraged to consider what strategies they might employ to increase the benefits at the next session. Some clients prefer to turn the volume up high during periods of severe pain, while others maintain it at a low level to ensure that they keep in tune with external events.

Changes in volume, attention to breathing, and variations in rhythm and tempo, plus the addition or deletion of movements such as toe or finger tapping, have been suggested and used successfully by clients.

Nursing's Role

The use of music requires some equipment, such as a portable cassette player and audio tape that may already be owned by the client or that may be easily obtained. It can be readily explained to clients and family members and mechanisms for its use (place, time, a quiet setting) easily arranged.

Distraction

Mechanisms of Action

Distraction means simply focusing attention on stimuli other than the pain sensation. This technique may increase pain tolerance or raise the perception threshold. Distraction places pain at the periphery of awareness so that the client can "tune out" the pain for the time distraction is being used. Whatever the exact mechanism may be, distraction does not make the pain disappear but makes it more tolerable.

Clinical Uses and Precautions

One of the most frequently used distraction techniques involves breathing exercises. The use of breathing exercises combines the benefits of relaxation with the effectiveness of distraction. Slow, deep abdominal breathing is an easily learned and useful approach. The client is directed to focus on his or her breathing by concentrating on the inhalations and exhalations. Breathing techniques must be carefully explained and monitored during the learning process so that the client does not breathe too rapidly (not to exceed 1 breath per second) or too deeply. When teaching breathing techniques, the nurse should ensure that the exhalation phase is passive and relaxed, rather than forced.

Like all techniques, some disadvantages are associated with distraction. Others may doubt the existence or severity of pain if distraction is a successful intervention. However, the very fact that distraction works indicates that pain is present and has been only temporarily relieved. Distraction is fatiguing and therefore is most useful for brief periods (less than 2 hours). Distraction requires energy and concentration, which results in a return of pain, irritability, and fatigue after its termination. However, the many benefits of distraction far outweigh the disadvantages, and an explanation of its efficacy and rationale should be provided to all clients in pain and their caregivers and family members.

Guidelines for Use

The types of distraction possible are limited only by the client's or the nurse's creativity and ingenuity. Methods include rhythmic breathing, rocking, singing or humming, describing pictures or photos aloud, listening to music, and playing games. Humor is a highly successful distraction strategy that has been shown to improve the release of the body's natural endorphins.

Nursing's Role

Distraction is one area of pain management that particularly highlights the creativity of the nurse in combination with the abilities and preferences of the client. While striving to suggest pleasant activities on which to focus, the nurse is also intent on giving the client a sense of personal control over the situation. One of the rewards of the successful choice of a distraction strategy is the true collaborative process that precedes it. The nurse also needs to focus on making sure that the other members of the health care team are aware of the mechanisms of distraction and especially that they know that the use of distraction does not mean that pain no longer exists. Rather, distraction has improved pain tolerance and temporarily made the qualities of the pain more acceptable to the client. The nurse may suggest that an analgesic be administered at the completion of the distraction exercise to encourage rest and comfort.

Positive Suggestion

Mechanisms of Action

Positive suggestion as used here refers to the administration of any type of analgesia in combination with an explanation of its potential positive effects. As with many other nonpharmacological forms of pain management, the involved mechanisms are not fully understood.

Clinical Uses

Placebos are traditionally used in clinical trials as a control against which to judge the efficacy of other analgesics. Evidence has shown that in a variety of painful conditions a remarkably constant proportion (about one third) of clients obtain significant relief from placebos. Disorders that have responded to placebos include pain associated with primary dysmenorrhea, chronic headache and migraines, rheumatoid and degenerative forms of arthritis, peptic ulcer, angina (with no demonstrable coronary artery disease), and cancer. Several studies also suggest that severe, steady postoperative pain often responds to placebo treatment.

Guidelines for Use

The physical characteristics of an intervention (e.g., pill vs. injection), the environment in which it is given, and the client-clinician relationship all appear important in determining the degree of response. Therefore, health care workers need to recognize the potential benefits of incorporating a positive, reassuring manner in their routine practice, to maximize the success of all interventions.

Nursing's Role

Nurses are the health care workers who most frequently administer the various pain treatments. As such, the role they play in maximizing the effectiveness of these interventions through positive suggestion is crucial.

Twenty-Three Things You Can Do to Improve Pain Management in Your Setting*

1. Do a pain audit. The first step toward change is demonstrating that a problem exists.
2. Create an awareness of the status of pain management in your agency. Inform physicians, nursing staff, and administrators of the state of pain control and areas in need of improvement.
3. Designate an "expert nurse" as the consultant to colleagues on pain. Support that nurse in getting additional pain education and in becoming a "watchdog" for untreated pain.
4. Educate the physicians. Circulate articles, monographs, or audio tapes of interest. Work to sponsor a continuing medical education offering on pain management.
5. Adopt a uniform pain assessment tool for use during admission to the unit of any patient with pain as a significant problem.

*Creasia JL and Parker B: *Conceptual foundations of professional nursing practice,* St. Louis, 1991, Mosby-Year Book, Inc.

6. Adopt an ongoing system for pain assessment (e.g., a visual analog scale).

7. Establish standards of care. You do not accept uncontrolled infection rates, extravasations, and falls, so why accept uncontrolled pain?

8. Involve others in pain management. Develop an army of supporters, e.g., workers from physical therapy, occupational therapy, and social service and the client's pharmacist.

9. Educate your clients. Clients must know that pain is preventable and treatable. Pain management should become a consumer issue, and clients should not settle for unrelieved pain.

10. Involve families in every aspect of pain management. Family members can be the greatest asset to pain relief or the greatest barrier.

11. Develop a "bag of tricks" for non-drug pain management, e.g., music, video tapes for relaxation, heat and cold therapy, instructions for breathing exercises, and audio tapes for imagery or relaxation.

12. Educate other nurses about basic principles of pain management.

13. Distribute equianalgesic charts to all nurses. They are required nursing knowledge.

14. Develop a relationship with the client's pharmacist. Develop a pharmacy advocate for pain management.

15. Include pain management in new employee orientation.

16. Develop a pocket card for every nurse and include a pain assessment scale and equianalgesia guides.

17. Make pain management accessible. Does the client's pharmacy stock appropriate medications and doses of drugs? Promote the use of longer-acting analgesics.

18. Develop an expectation that PAIN CAN BE RELIEVED. The vast majority of nurses and clients believe that cancer pain is inevitable and uncontrollable.

19. Plan for continuity in pain management.

20. Document pain assessment. The client's pain experience must be effectively communicated among all disciplines involved.

21. Evaluate your efforts.

22. Ask the client. The client remains the best authority on his or her pain and our treatment of it.

23. Provide the kind of pain management that you would seek for your own family member.

Nursing Care for Musculoskeletal Disorders

Cast Care*

The First 24 Hours

Plaster casts need at least 24 hours to dry. Instruct clients to follow these rules:

- Avoid handling cast as much as possible.
- When the cast must be handled, as when changing body position, use only the palms and support the cast under the joint.
- Use a fan 18 to 24 inches from the cast to aid drying, exposing the entire cast.
- Do not cover cast with linen for first 24 hours.
- Keep cast and extremity above heart level for at least 48 hours.
- Put ice directly over the fractured area for 24 hours, but enclose ice in plastic to keep the cast dry.
- Move body parts above and below the cast regularly to aid circulation and relieve stiffness.
- Massage joints and extremities around cast to improve circulation.

General Cast Care

After the cast is set and completely dry, offer the client and caregiver these general guidelines for the duration of the cast's use:

- Do not walk on a leg cast for the first 48 hours.
- When ambulation is allowed on a cast, walk on the walking heel.
- If the arm is in a cast, use the sling for support.

Plaster Casts

- Keep plaster cast clean and dry at all times, covering it with plastic when bathing or going out in wet weather.
- The cast can be spot-cleaned with a damp cloth and scouring powder; brush crumbs from edges of the cast.

*From Mourad L: *Orthopedic disorders*, St. Louis, 1990, Mosby-Year Book, Inc.

Synthetic Casts

- Clients in synthetic casts may be allowed to bathe and swim, if there is no wound under the cast. However, the cast must be rinsed thoroughly inside and out after swimming.
- Dry synthetic casts and stockinettes thoroughly each time they get wet. Use a towel to blot the cast, then dry it with a hair dryer set on low. When the cast is not cold and damp to the touch, it is dry.
- When bathing, use only a small amount of mild soap around the synthetic cast, rinsing under the cast thoroughly.

Skin Care

- Do not insert objects under the cast; avoid scraping or adding pressure, thus causing infection or sores under the cast.
- Use powders and lotions only outside the cast so that the skin stays clean and soft. Powder inside a cast can cake and cause sore areas.
- Once the cast is removed, do not try to scrub away old skin cells all at once. Soften and condition the skin with a damp cloth and Woolite to loosen dead cells without injury. Gently wash skin with water and Woolite; keep Woolite on skin for 5 to 10 minutes; rinse thoroughly and pat dry; apply moisturizer. Repeat each day till skin is nearly normal.

After-Cast Care

- The affected part may be sore and weak for several days or longer. Limit use for 1 to 4 weeks until muscles are stronger.
- A mild pain medication may be needed for a day or two after removal to relieve the soreness of reuse.
- Elevate the part after cast removal for 1 to 3 days to relieve swelling.

Recovery After Total Hip Replacement

It is crucial that clients recovering from hip replacement maintain proper hip position during recovery; position the client to keep the hip from bending, using an abduction pillow to keep legs apart and prevent their turning inward. Providing appropriate precautions is particularly important since the hip will have limited range of motion and prostheses can slip out of position. Use the following guidelines for instructing client and caregiver on home recovery after total hip replacement (adapted from Mourad, 1990).

Safety Considerations

- Legs and ankles should not be crossed while standing, sitting, or lying.
- In a seated position, feet should be 6 inches apart, and knees should be below hips (sitting on a pillow aids in maintaining this position).
- The client must be cautioned not to bend at the waist; a long-handled shoehorn and a reacher should be used.
- Crutches, and later a cane, should be used to avoid putting excess weight on the new hip.
- Aid balance by:
  - Using handrails
  - Wearing low-heeled shoes
  - Ensuring that floors are free of water, wax, and objects that can interfere with balance
- When car travel is allowed (approximately 3 months after surgery), it is important for the client to stop every hour and walk several minutes to increase leg circulation.

Post-Surgery Exercises

It is usually recommended that each exercise be repeated 5 to 10 times, twice a day, as prescribed. Instruct the client as follows:

- Lie flat on the back and lift affected leg straight off the bed about 12 inches. Hold for 5 seconds, then relax.
- Sit with feet on the floor and lift affected knee straight off the chair about 4 inches. Hold for 5 seconds, then relax.
- Lie on unaffected side with a pillow between the knees. Try to lift the affected leg straight off the pillow. Hold for 5 seconds, then relax.

The following exercises should be done while the client is standing and holding onto something stable. As a rule, the client will be prescribed to repeat each 5 to 10 times, twice daily, or as ordered by the physician.

- Bend affected leg and bring up toward chest; do not exceed a 90-degree angle. Straighten leg again.
- Point hips, knees, and feet straight in front. Slowly move the affected leg out to the side and then back again to the other leg.
- Bend the knee and move the leg backward without arching the back. Return the leg to the starting position.

In addition to these exercises, as soon as the physician or physical therapist prescribes, the client should make walking a part of the daily routine, beginning with 10 minutes 3 times a day, and working up to 30 minutes once a day.

Recovery After Total Knee Replacement

Teach both the client and caregiver to monitor for and notify the physician of any of the following signs:

- Increased knee pain
- Swelling in the leg or knee
- Unusual or increased pain in the knee
- Fluid leakage from the incision
- Shortness of breath or chest pain
- Pain or swelling of the calf muscle in either lower leg

Strengthening and Range-of-Motion Exercises

Introduce and monitor the following exercises, for strengthening and increasing mobility, only as they are prescribed by the physician or physical therapist (adapted from Mourad, 1990):

- Assume a supine position in bed with a towel under the ankle. Push affected knee down into the mattress. Hold for 5 seconds, then relax. Repeat 6 times.
- Assume a supine position in bed with a towel under the ankle. Push the heel down into the mattress. Hold for 5 seconds, then relax. Repeat 6 times.
- Assume a supine position in bed. Slide the heel of the affected leg back toward the buttocks while bending the knee. Hold for 5 seconds. Repeat 6 times.
- Assume a supine position. While tightening the thigh muscles, lift the affected leg about 12 inches. Hold for 5 to 10 seconds. Slowly lower the leg. Repeat with other leg. Do 6 times for each leg.
- From a seated position, slowly raise the foot, then bring it back under the chair as far as possible. Repeat with the other leg. Do 6 times for each leg.

Crutch Walking

The guidelines below may be shared with clients who have been prescribed to use crutches. In addition to these guidelines, caution clients to avoid slick floors and throw rugs and to keep the crutch tips clean and in good condition to avoid slipping (adapted from Mourad, 1990).

Walking: Some weight borne on both legs

Move one leg and the opposite crutch forward at the same time; then move the other crutch and opposite leg forward. Continue to move one crutch and the opposite leg forward with each step.

Walking: No weight borne on one leg

Put all weight on unaffected foot and leg. Move both crutches and affected leg forward about 8 to 10 inches. Shift weight to wrists and hands and step forward with unaffected leg. Rest, if needed, then continue in the same pattern. Always move the crutches and the foot in the cast forward at the same time.

Walking: One foot or leg in cast

Always keep casted foot in front of the other foot when using crutches to prevent tripping, catching cast, or aggravating the injury by putting more weight on the foot than allowed.

Sitting down in a chair

Walk up close to chair. Turn, then back up until chair touches the back of the knees. Hold the handgrips of both crutches with one hand, and with the other hand reach for the arm or seat of the chair. Sink into the chair by bearing weight on the crutches' handgrips and the chair arm. Slide affected leg forward while sitting.

Getting up from a chair

Place both crutches on one side. Put one hand on top of both handgrips and put the other hand on the chair arm or seat. Push up from the chair to a standing position. Place a crutch under each arm. Be sure the chair is strong and sturdy enough.

Going up stairs with crutch in each hand

Walk up close to the bottom step. Put all weight on the handgrips and step up to the next step with the unaffected leg and foot. Then bring the body, affected leg, and crutches up to the same step. Be sure crutches are centered on the step.

Going down stairs with crutch in each hand

Walk up near the edge of the top step. Bend hips and place both crutches and affected leg on next lower step. Put weight on crutches and bring unaffected leg down to the same step. Continue down the stairs in the same way.

Going up stairs using a bannister

Walk up close to the stairs. Place both crutches under the arm opposite the bannister and grasp both handgrips. Grasp the bannister with the free hand. Put all weight on the hands and lift unaffected foot and leg up to the next step. Bring the crutches, body, and affected leg up to the same step. Continue up the stairs in the same way.

Going down stairs using a bannister

Put both crutches in one hand, holding them together at the handgrips and under the arm. Put the other hand on the bannister. Move the affected leg and crutches down to the next step, but do not put any weight on the affected leg if it is to bear no weight. Put all weight on the hands and wrists on the crutches and bannister and step down with the unaffected leg. Continue down the stairs in the same way.

Stopping to rest on crutches

Rest without leaning shoulders on the crutches' shoulder pads. Leaning too long or putting too much pressure in the axillary area can injure the nerves and cut off arm circulation. Instead, put the weight on wrists, handgrips, and unaffected leg, and hold crutches nearer the chest. Tingling and numbness in the arm indicate too much pressure on the axillary area.

Traction

Clients in traction who can be cared for at home include infants needing divarication traction, clients needing several weeks of balanced-suspension traction, and individuals with external fixation devices in place. The client in traction usually needs a family member or other person who is willing, available, and able to learn how to care for the client. This person must also understand the traction application and be able to provide all custodial care.

The two types of traction are skin traction and skeletal traction. Only skin traction is used in the home. Skeletal traction must be done in a hospital and must remain in continuous use until the physician determines that it can be removed, usually when bone healing has occurred or when surgical repairs are done so that healing can continue at home and out of traction.

Skin traction is used to treat muscle injuries, bone fractures, ruptured or herniated discs, muscle contractures, and arthritic conditions. It can be applied to an arm, the head, a leg, or the pelvis. Skin traction is applied to the skin surfaces, usually by a pelvic belt, head halter, traction boot, or moleskin straps covered with elastic wraps. It is attached to ropes and weights appropriate to the age and condition of the client (Mourad, 1990).

Initial Needs Assessment for Traction in the Home Setting[*]

The following areas of client need should be assessed and the findings incorporated into the care plan:

- How will the client manage the activities of daily living, such as eating, toileting, bathing, dressing, and, if allowed, transferring from bed to chair or bed to standing position?
- How will the client's change in activity affect his or her nutritional and metabolic needs?
- Will the client be able to perform range-of-motion exercises with the unaffected extremities?
- How will the client and family adjust to continued needs and interruption in their usual lifestyle?
- Are there other client needs related to health issues such as diabetes, cardiovascular disease, or traumatic injuries?
- Will the client need ongoing laboratory tests, such as those for managing anticoagulant therapy?
- How will the client get to the physician's office for follow-up care?
- Do the client and significant other understand the signs and symptoms of potential complications related to traction application?
- Is there a family member or significant other who can provide the necessary care for the client? How much assistance does the family need for personal care, meals, and monitoring the client's progress?
- Does the client have a skilled care need that can be met only by a licensed practitioner (e.g., skeletal traction set-up, a pin site that needs care, skin breakdown, a change in metabolic or cardiovascular status)?

*Folcik MA, Carini-Garcia G, and Birmingham JJ: *Traction: Assessment and management*, St. Louis, 1994, Mosby-Year Book, Inc.

- Does the client have medical insurance that will help pay for needed services? Has the insurance company been contacted to determine whether home care services are covered?
- Is the client's home environment conducive to recovery (e.g., easy access in and out of the house, bathroom convenient to the client, phone for emergency use)?
- Will the client need a special bed for the application of traction, and does it fit in the client's home?
- Does the client know how to do pin site care, and are there supplies for the procedure?
- Will the client be able to resume the instrumental activities of daily living (IADL), such as telephoning and managing money affairs?

Nursing Care Plan for the Client in Traction

The client's individualized plan of care should address the following points:

- The client's diagnosis, including the reason for traction
- The rehabilitation potential and short- and long-term goals
- The client's needs and any potential problems in meeting those needs
- Problems associated with the family support system
- Types and frequency of services to be provided, including medication administration, nutrition needs, procedures, equipment, and transportation
- Functional limitations of the client, particularly regarding ambulation
- Safety measures to protect the client from complications and additional injury
- Psychosocial needs of the client, especially those related to the interruption of work, school, or other social activities
- Client and family education

The care plan should include the following points:

- Observing the client and family in skin care, equipment safety, pin site care, nutrition planning, fluid and electrolyte balance, signs of complications and the need for follow-up medical care, and medication compliance
- Monitoring skin care
- Monitoring bowel and bladder function
- Assisting in obtaining laboratory studies for the client who is on anticoagulant therapy
- Observing ROM exercises for all joints
- Assessing the client for symptoms of other diseases or the exacerbation of existing diseases

- Assisting the client and family with stress and coping strategies
- Coordinating all care being rendered to the client, including that provided by the orthopaedic surgeon, other physicians (surgeons, cardiologists, endocrinologists), other health professionals, and the family or significant others

Implementation Strategies for Skin Traction[*]

- Look over all areas of the skin where the traction is to be applied. The traction will pull on the skin and could cause additional injury to already compromised skin. It should not be applied over open sores, rashes, bruises, marked swelling, or raised moles or warts.
- Do not shave the skin under the areas where the traction is to be applied. Shaving could cause small cuts that could become inflamed under the traction.
- Make sure the skin is clean and dry to prevent chafing or maceration caused by excess water on the skin.
- Provide the client and family with written instructions on equipment and its application, along with phone numbers of the agency, the ordering physician, and the equipment supplier.
- Ensure that the client and caregiver understand exactly when and if the weights can be removed at times—especially at night. The physician may give an order that the client can be in 2 hours, then out 2 hours, and off at night. Being in traction at night often prevents that client from relaxing muscles to allow rest and sleep.
- Usually the client will receive relief of muscle spasms and pain from the effects of the traction. If the spasms or pain increase, however, be sure to notify the physician. Adjustments in the amount of weights, positions, or time in traction may be needed for benefits to be achieved. At times, the use of traction may need to be stopped if there are adverse reactions.
- Teach the client how to count arterial pulses in the extremities or area in traction; how to feel for temperature, color, and swelling; and how to wrap elastic bandages (if used) properly to prevent overtightness leading to more swelling, numbness or tingling, or throbbing under the bandages. Elastic bandages should be removed and reapplied more loosely if these symptoms occur after the traction has been applied.

[*]From Mourad L: *Orthopedic disorders*, St. Louis, 1990, Mosby-Year Book, Inc.

Death and Dying: Information for Families Concerning Imminent Death

The following information can answer questions and concerns families and caregivers have when caring for an individual who is dying.*

Signs of Approaching Death

- The arms and legs of the client may become cool to the touch, and you may notice the underside of the client's body becoming much darker in color. These are signs of blood circulation slowing down.
- The client will gradually spend more and more time sleeping during the day and at times will be difficult to arouse. This sign is a result of a change in the body's metabolism.
- The client may become increasingly confused about time, place, and identity of close and familiar people. Again, this is a result of change in body metabolism.
- Incontinence (loss of control) of urine and bowel movements may become a problem during the final days.
- Oral secretions may become more profuse and collect in the back of the throat. You may have heard friends refer to a "death rattle." This sign is a result of the client's inability to cough up normal saliva.
- Clarity of hearing and vision decrease slightly.
- You may notice the client becoming restless, pulling at bed linen, and having visions of people or things that do not exist. These signs are a result of a decrease in the oxygen circulation to the brain and a change in body metabolism.
- The client will have decreased desire for food and drink because the body will naturally begin to conserve energy that would otherwise be expended in eating and drinking.
- During sleep, at first, you will notice the client's breathing patterns changing to an irregular pace and there may be 10- to 30-second periods of no breathing. Your physician and nurse refer to this as periods of "apnea." This sign is common

*Developed by the Seattle/King County Visiting Nurse Services, Seattle, Wash.

and indicates a decrease in circulation and a buildup of waste products in the blood.

- You will notice that the amount of urine will decrease as death grows near.

What To Do About These Signs

- Keep warm blankets on the client to prevent him or her from feeling too cold. Electric blankets should be used with caution so that burns do not occur.
- Plan your times with the client for occasions when he or she seems most alert.
- Remind the client frequently about what day it is, what time it is, who is in the room, and who is talking.
- Consult with your nurse about obtaining pads to place under the incontinent client and other techniques to ensure cleanliness.
- If and when oral secretions build up, elevating the head of the bed with pillows will make breathing easier.
- Ice chips and cool, moist wash cloths will relieve feelings of dehydration.
- Keep lights on in the room when vision decreases, and never assume that the client cannot hear you. Hearing is the last of the five senses to be lost.
- Talk calmly and assuredly with a confused person so as not to startle or frighten him or her.

Appendices

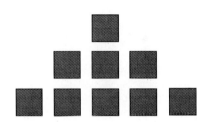

Appendix A: Key Home Health Care Definitions and Roles

Case management: The supervision of the care given to a specific client or caseload population. In home health care, this is often a primary care model with the RN case manager rendering the skilled care, supervising, or collaborating with other ordered professional services. Communication among the services and disciplines involved in the care must be documented in the clinical record. In these care conferences, input is given to the RN case manager to assist the "intradisciplinary" team in reaching the client's goals.

Chaplaincy services: The chaplain serves a population that spans the life continuum from birth through death. The chaplain, like the professional nurse, interacts with clients and their families and friends at some of the most difficult times of their lives. This struggle with the meaning of life, experienced by many who have significant health concerns, is the work of the chaplain, regardless of any formal religious beliefs. The role varies, based on the setting, the client and family, or other needs. It may include bereavement counseling, serving on ethics committees, hospice staff support, or performing the sacrament of the sick. The chaplain facilitates the client's movement toward his or her own resolution of life's questions.

Clients who may benefit from chaplaincy services include those for whom the NANDA nursing diagnosis *spiritual distress* (distress of the human spirit) has been identified as an appropriate nursing diagnosis. Other clients may have a need for spiritual care based on their health problems. For example, the elderly client, who is temporarily homebound because of a recent fall and fracture and misses going to church services on Sunday morning, may need a call made to his or her priest or minister to arrange visits to his or her home.

Daily care: Medicare clients meet eligibility requirements when skilled nursing care is needed 4 or fewer days per week. This is regardless of the duration of the care. For the purposes of qualifying a Medicare client for home health services, daily is defined as 5 or more days per week. When nursing care is needed 5, 6, or 7 days per week (daily), eligibility is established only when the service is not needed indefinitely. This means that the home care nurse needs a projected endpoint for daily visits. These clients who need daily nursing care for an unspecified amount of time or indefinitely do not receive coverage under Medicare.

Insulin administration is the exception to daily intermittent care. In unusual circumstances, where the client is physically or mentally unable to self-inject and there is no available able and willing caregiver, the HHA can give these visits daily, while trying to locate a caregiver. These are the only daily visits that usually do not need a projected ending date.

Dietitian: The role of the professional, registered dietitian in home care is expanding as more clients are cared for in the community setting. Many home health agencies and hospices have professional dietitians available to make home visits and provide consultative services to promote optimal client nutrition. Another important component of the dietitian's role is as in-service educator for the home health and hospice team.

Often, after being hospitalized, clients will receive instructions on nutrition in relation to their unique needs and medical condition. Some of the common reasons for consultation with a dietitian are enteral/parenteral nutrition, diabetes, AIDS, and other chronic diseases, as well as assessment and monitoring of nutritional needs. Malnutrition in the elderly is also a concern of the professional dietitian.

More innovative insurers are reimbursing for this care if the HHA can clearly articulate the client's need and justify the visits as part of the comprehensive plan.

Enterostomal therapy (ET) nurse: Some HHAs have an ET nurse available to their nurses as a consultant and clinical specialist. This role is particularly important in the HHA and in hospice settings with a high volume of clients with ostomy and wound problems. The clinical specialist role is also important in that the educational needs of the clinical visiting staff and community are served.

Evaluation visit (assessment visit): This is the first or initial home visit to determine whether the client meets the HHA's criteria for admission. It is often the first skilled visit, made when the nurse already has specific physician's orders and is providing a skilled service.

Homebound: Synonymous with *confined primarily to the home as a result of medical reasons,* the term connotes that it is a "considerable and taxing effort" to leave the home.

Home health aide (HHA): The HHA's primary, supportive function is to provide personal care and ADL assistance. This role and the associated functions are very important. The HHA usually spends more actual time with the client and family than any other team member. The HHA's contribution is invaluable to both the team process and positive client outcomes.

Hospice care: Hospice care focuses on the comfort and quality of life to assist the terminally ill client and family to make every remaining day the best that it can be. Hospice is a philosophy and can be provided in any setting, such as home or an inpatient hospice unit. Palliative care, emotional support, and control of pain and other symptoms are some of the areas of expertise addressed by the hospice team. Through team meetings and individual visits, the physician, the spiritual counselor, the primary nurse, the hospice volunteers, the social worker, the hospice clinical specialist, and others assist the client and family in meeting their unique needs.

After death, bereavement support services are provided to the family as a key component of continued hospice care.

Management and Evaluation of the Client Plan of Care (POC): This Medicare service is called various things, including skilled management, skilled planning and assessment, skilled management and planning, case management, and M and E of the client POC.

Before this became a covered service by Medicare, nurses practicing in home health had limited exposure to this level of care. Many times clients were kept on the service by HHAs with no reimbursement because the client had an extensive medical history of multifaceted problems, no caregivers, or multiple needs that the caregiver could not safely and effectively meet. However, they were frequently readmitted when they fell and refractured their hip or had an acute exacerbation of CHF or COPD that necessitated hospitalization.

In discussing this skilled service, the Medicare manual states: "Skilled nursing . . . where underlying conditions or complications require that only a registered nurse can ensure that essential nonskilled care is achieving its purpose. . . . The complexity of the necessary unskilled services which are a necessary part of the medical treatment must require the involvement of skilled nursing personnel to promote the client's recovery and medical safety in view of the beneficiary's overall condition."

The following are typical issues that need to be addressed when determining if the client is appropriate for management. Evaluation and documentation may support these services: (1) the client's medical history; (2) the caregiver's support system; (3) current or highly probable medical concerns, based on past history; (4) multiple medications listed on the POC; (5) functional limitations that affect care; (6) safety or other high-risk factors identified; (7) unusual home/environment; (8) ordered disciplines and interventions; (9) diagnoses and underlying pathologies that affect the plan; and (10) the client's mental status. The nurse needs to assess and document why the skills of an RN are needed to promote the client's recovery (document evidence of movement toward client goals) and ensure medical safety.

Medical Social Services (MSS): The social services used in home health care are directly related to the treatment of the client's medical condition. When social concerns impede the effective implementation of the POC, a social worker is appropriate. The social problems seen in home health care include finances, housing, and caregiver concerns. The services must be documented to focus on the client, even though the social worker also assists the family, in conjunction with the client in home health care.

Occupational therapy (OT): OT assists the client to attain the maximum level of physical and psychosocial independence. Areas of expertise include fine motor coordination, perceptual-motor skills, sensory testing, adaptive/assistive equipment, ADL, and specialized upper extremity/hand therapies. The kinds of problems frequently seen in home health care which require OT include CVAs, amputations, and lung processes for conservation of energy skills. For Medicare clients, OT is not a qualifying skilled service that can begin home health care services. However, when a client has already been receiving another skilled service, such as nursing or physical therapy, and the client no longer needs these services, the occupational therapist can continue to provide continued services.

Occupational Safety and Health Administration (OSHA): Nurses have heard much in recent years about the need for the practice of universal precautions. The Labor Department's OSHA released its final rule to prevent occupational transmission of bloodborne pathogens and infections. Nurses are well aware of the dangers of hepatitis B and HIV. Employees must create infection control policies that support universal precautions. In addition, nurses, home health aides, and other staff members must be educated about the policy. In practice, this means that hepatitis B immunizations are available when the job requires exposure to blood or other potentially infectious body fluids. The HHA must also provide protective equipment and supplies. This includes gloves, face masks or other protective shields, aprons that are fluidproof, gowns, and other needed protection. These should be provided by the agency free of charge to the home care nurses and staff. There are also guidelines on blood or other body fluid transport, blood spill clean-up, and the safe disposal of infectious waste.

Personal emergency response systems (PERS): These systems represent a unique technology that links the frail or elderly with community resources, neighbors, or a friend at the push of a button or through voice-activated mechanisms. Although there are different types, all are telephone-service dependent. PERS may be appropriate for single clients returning home after surgery, clients who live alone or spend many hours at home alone, or clients at risk from falls. PERS signal for help at the push of a button, which is worn by the PERS subscriber. For the system to be effective, the emergency device must be worn at all times. Home care and hospice nurses are in a unique position to identify this safety need in the community setting, so a referral can be initiated.

Pharmacist: The role of the clinical pharmacist in home care is growing, as the emphasis on quality and addressing client needs from an "intradisciplinary" model continues. In practice, nurses are acutely aware of many clients who are inappropriately or overmedicated. It is the nurse in the community who sees the whole picture and the shoeboxes full of medications given to clients from multiple physicians. It is in this instance that the nurse addresses safety concerns, acts as the client's advocate, and consults with the pharmacist who can effectively evaluate the multiple medication regimens.

Traditionally, the pharmacist has been considered the provider of a product—drugs. While this is certainly true, there are many services that the pharmacist can offer to the home care team.

Many, if not most, home care clients are elderly and have multiple risk factors for therapeutic misadventures, secondary to drug therapy. They may have multiple pathologies and different prescribers, exhibit polypharmacy (both prescription and nonprescription medications), and are at a greater risk for adverse effects from medications due to altered physiology, secondary to aging and disabilities (e.g., poor eyesight, impaired hearing, arthritic fingers). Don't forget that a pharmacist can offer more than the provision of drugs: the pharmacist is the drug expert. This discipline is in an excellent position to review medication regimens and screen for drug interactions (drug-drug, drug-disease, drug-food), adverse drug reactions, and incorrect doses or dosage forms and to make recommendations. The pharmacist can suggest simplifying the client's medication regimen, by altering drug delivery systems and medication administration scheduling or by suggesting how to monitor and assess the therapeutic or toxic effect of drugs. Home care providers can always turn to a pharmacist for drug information, for inservice education, or for participation in case conferences and home care/hospice rounds.

Physical therapy (PT): PT services usually are based on client need and diagnosis. PT, like OT and S-LP, should have a restorative function. This usually means that the client has a good or fair rehabilitation potential. The PT documentation must show progression toward a goal. The most common kinds of client problems in home health care which require PT include CVAs, hip fractures or surgery, knee replacements, and acute exacerbations of osteoarthritis. One of the primary PT skills focuses on teaching the client and family the home exercise regimens.

Psychiatric nurse: The role of the psychiatric nurse in home care has been expanding as more care is provided in the community setting. With the Medicare manual revision of 1989, the role of the psychiatric nurse was clarified to assist the agency in obtaining payment for clients that meet the criteria for coverage. The kinds of problems seen in home care by specially trained psychiatric nurses include depression and therapy, bipolar disorder, and evaluation of medication therapeutic levels and effectiveness, as well as many geriatric affective disorders.

The social worker may also be involved in counseling, while the psychiatric nurse is primarily needed for the skills of medication evaluation, observation and assessment, and evaluation and therapy.

Sometimes, it may be appropriate for cases to be shared. The psychiatric nurse visit, which is a skilled nursing visit, may be covered for that expertise. For example, the client with medical-surgical problems and depression or manipulative behavior may also be seen by the psychiatric nurse, the same way the primary nurse may arrange for the ET nurse to see a client with specialized wound problems. The psychiatric nurse would set up the POC in conjunction with the primary nurse and other team members to establish a behavioral plan for the team. The documentation needs to focus on the psychiatric needs, as documented by the psychiatric data base, such as a mental status exam and other interventions.

Rehabilitative services: In home health care, rehabilitative services include the services of PT, OT, and speech/language therapy, all of which should be restorative in focus. When any of these services are indicated, based on client need, diagnosis, and client rehabilitation potential status, there must be sufficient documentation of communication among all services. This multidisciplinary case conferencing should be reflected in the progress notes at least every 4 to 6 weeks.

Skilled nursing: Skilled nursing occurs when an RN uses knowledge as a professional nurse to execute skills, render judgments, and evaluate process and outcome. If a nonprofessional can perform a particular function, it is probably not a skilled function. Teaching, assessment, and evaluation skills are some of the many areas of expertise that are classified as skilled services. As the length of inpatient facility stays have decreased, so has the amount of teaching before discharge. To justify teaching visits, always document and describe specific knowledge deficits that are assessed on admission. Explain that client teaching was incomplete or was not effective in the inpatient setting. For example, a client discharged from the hospital on April 2 began a new medication regimen on April 1. Admission to home health care would evaluate the medication effectiveness; however, the dates should be documented clearly to justify medication effectiveness and teaching visits.

Speech-language pathology (S-LP): S-LP services are a vital rehabilitative service indicated for various speech pathologies. Clients that frequently need home health S-LP services have the following problems: CVAs, tracheostomy, laryngectomy, and various neuromuscular diseases. Progress must be noted in the clinical documentation, and case conferencing must occur. It is important that the reason for homebound status be clearly and regularly identified in the clinical record.

Supervisory visit: A supervisory visit at least every 2 weeks (484.36) is a Condition of Participation in the Medicare program. This is not a covered service and may be an administrative expense. A supervisory visit becomes billable when a skilled service is performed during the same visit. For example, a bedridden client has a decubitus ulcer and the nurse changes the dressing after observing the HHA completing the bed/bath and reviewing the HHA assignment sheet.

Adapted from Marrelli TM: *Handbook of home health standards and documentation guidelines for reimbursement, ed. 2,* St. Louis, 1994, Mosby-Year Book, Inc.

Appendix B: Key Home Health Care Abbreviations

The following abbreviations are among those most commonly used in the practice of home care. Please refer to your agency's own designated list of approved abbreviations for daily use in documentation.

ADL	Activities of daily living
ALS	Amyotrophic lateral sclerosis (Lou Gehrig's disease)
AMI	Acute myocardial infarction
APHA	American Public Health Association
ASCVD	Arteriosclerotic cardiovascular disease
ASD	Atrial septal defect
ASHD	Arteriosclerotic heart disease
BP	Blood pressure
BPH	Benign prostatic hypertrophy
BRP	Bathroom privileges
BS	Blood sugar
CA	Cancer
CABG	Coronary artery bypass graft
CBC	Complete blood count
CDC	Centers for Disease Control and Prevention
CHF	Congestive heart failure
CNS	Clinical nurse specialist
COPD	Chronic obstructive pulmonary disease
COPS	(Medicare) Conditions of Participation
CPM	Continuous passive motion
CPR	Cardiopulmonary resuscitation
C/S	Cesarean section
CVA	Cerebral vascular accident
CXR	Chest x ray
DJD	Degenerative joint disease
DM	Diabetes mellitus
DOE	Dyspnea on exertion
DRG	Diagnosis Related Group
DX	Diagnosis
EDC	Estimated date of confinement
ET	Enterostomal therapist
FBS	Fasting blood sugar
FHR	Fetal heart rate
FX	Fracture

HCFA	Health Care Financing Administration
HEP	Home exercise prograrn
HHA	Home health agency or Home health aide
HHC	Home health care
HIM	Health Insurance Manual
HME	Home medical equipment
HVGS	High voltage galvanic stimulation
IDDM	Insulin dependent diabetes mellitus
IM	Intramuscular
IPPB	Intermittent positive pressure breathing
IV	Intravenous
JCAHO	Joint Commission on Accreditation of Healthcare Organizations
LLE	Left lower extremity
LLL	Left lower lung
LUE	Left upper extremity
MI	Myocardial infarction
MOW	Meals on Wheels
MSS	Medical Social Services
NHP	Nursing home placement
NIDDM	Non-insulin dependent diabetes mellitus
NIH	National Institutes of Health
OBS	Organic brain syndrome
OSHA	Occupational Safety and Health Administration
OT	Occupational therapy
PCA	Patient-controlled analgesia
PERLA	Pupils equal, react to light and accommodation
PICC (line)	Peripherally inserted central catheter
PKU	Phenylketonuria
PO	By mouth (orally)
POC	Plan of care
PRE	Progressive resistive exercises
PRN	As needed
PT	Physical therapy
PVD	Peripheral vascular disease
RHHI	Regional Home Health Intermediary
RLE	Right lower extremity
RLL	Right lower lung
ROM	Range of motion
RUE	Right upper extremity
S-LP	Speech-language pathology
SNV	Skilled nursing visit
SOB	Shortness of breath
S/P	Status post

SQ	Subcutaneous
SX	Symptoms
TENS	Transcutaneous electrical nerve stimulation
TIA	Transient ischemic attack
Title XVIII	The Medicare section of the Social Security Act
Title XIX	The Medicaid section of the Social Security Act
Title XX	The Social Services section of the Social Security Act
TKR	Total knee replacement
TO	Telephone order
TPN	Total parenteral nutrition
TPR	Temperature, pulse, and respiration
TUR	Transurethral resection
TURP	Transurethral resection of prostate
TX	Treatment
UA/C&S	Urinalysis/culture and sensitivity
UE	Upper extremity
URI	Upper respiratory infection
UTI	Urinary tract infection
VO	Verbal order
WIC	Women, Infants, and Children Program
WNL	Within normal limits

From Marrelli TM: *Handbook of home health standards and documentation guidelines for reimbursement, ed. 2*, St. Louis, 1994, Mosby-Year Book, Inc.

Appendix C: NANDA-Approved Nursing Diagnoses

Activity intolerance
Activity intolerance, high risk for
Adjustment, impaired
Airway clearance, ineffective
Anxiety
Aspiration, high risk for
Body image disturbance
Body temperature, altered, high risk for
Bowel elimination, altered
Bowel incontinence
Breast-feeding, effective
Breast-feeding, ineffective
Breast-feeding, interrupted
Breathing pattern, ineffective
Cardiac output, decreased
Caregiver role strain
Caregiver role strain, high risk for
Comfort, altered
Communication, impaired verbal
Constipation
Constipation, colonic
Constipation, perceived
Coping, defensive
Coping, family: potential for growth
Coping, ineffective family: compromised
Coping, ineffective family: disabling
Coping, ineffective individual
Decisional conflict (specify)
Denial, ineffective
Diarrhea
Disuse syndrome, high risk for
Diversional activity deficit
Dysreflexia
Family processes, altered
Fatigue
Fear
Fluid volume deficit (1)
Fluid volume deficit (2)
Fluid volume deficit, high risk for

Fluid volume excess
Gas exchange, impaired
Grieving, anticipatory
Grieving, dysfunctional
Growth and development, altered
Health maintenance, altered
Health seeking behaviors (specify)
Home maintenance management, impaired
Hopelessness
Hyperthermia
Hypothermia
Incontinence, bowel
Incontinence, functional
Incontinence, reflex
Incontinence, stress
Incontinence, total
Incontinence, urge
Infant feeding pattern, ineffective
Infection, high risk for
Injury, high risk for
Knowledge deficit (specify)
Management of therapeutic regimen (individual), ineffective
Mobility, impaired physical
Noncompliance (specify)
Nutrition, altered: less than body requirements
Nutrition, altered: more than body requirements
Nutrition, altered: high risk for more than body requirements
Oral mucous membrane, altered
Pain
Pain, chronic
Parental role conflict
Parenting, altered
Parenting, altered, high risk for
Peripheral neurovascular dysfunction, high risk for
Personal identity disturbance
Poisoning, high risk for
Post-trauma response
Powerlessness
Protection, altered
Rape-trauma syndrome
Rape-trauma syndrome: compound reaction
Rape-trauma syndrome: silent reaction
Relocation stress syndrome
Role performance, altered

Self-care deficit: bathing/hygiene
Self-care deficit: dressing/grooming
Self-care deficit: feeding
Self-care deficit: toileting
Self-concept, disturbance in
Self-esteem disturbance
Self-esteem, chronic low
Self-esteem, situational low
Self-mutilation, high risk for
Sensory/perceptual alterations (specify) (visual, auditory, kinesthetic, gustatory, tactile, olfactory)
Sexual dysfunction
Sexuality patterns, altered
Skin integrity, impaired
Skin integrity, impaired, high risk for
Sleep pattern disturbance
Social interaction, impaired
Social isolation
Spiritual distress (distress of the human spirit)
Suffocation, high risk for
Swallowing, impaired
Thermoregulation, ineffective
Thought processes, altered
Tissue integrity, impaired
Tissue perfusion, altered (specify) (renal, cerebral, cardiopulmonary, gastrointestinal, peripheral)
Trauma, high risk for
Unilateral neglect
Urinary elimination, altered patterns
Urinary retention
Ventilation, inability to sustain spontaneous
Ventilatory weaning process, dysfunctional (DVWR)
Violence, high risk for: self-directed or directed at others

Appendix D: Selected Common Laboratory Values

Test	Conventional Range	SI Range
BLOOD		
Acetoacetate plus acetone	Negative	
Aldolase	1.3-8.2 U/L	22-137 nmol sec^{-1}/L
Ammonia	12-55 µmol/L	12-55 µmol/L
Amylase	4-25 units/ml	4-25 arb. units
Arterial blood gases		
CO_2 content	24-30 mEq/L	
pH	7.35-7.45	Same
PCO_2	35-45 mm Hg	4.7-6.0 kPa
PO_2	75-100 mm Hg (age dependent in room air)	10.0-13.3 kPa
BUN	8-25 mg/100 ml	
Bilirubin	Direct: up to 0.4 mg/100 ml; total: up to 1.0 mg/100 ml Indirect: up to 1.0 mg/100 ml	Up to 7 µmol/L
Calcium	8.5-10.5 mg/100 ml	2.1-2.6 mmol/L
Chloride	100-106 mEq/L	100-106 mmol/L
Complement, total hemolytic	150-250 U/ml	
C3	83-177 mg/100 ml	0.83-1.77 g/L
C4	15-45 mg/100 ml	0.15-0.45 g/L
Complete blood count		
Hematocrit	Female: 37%-48% Male: 45%-52%	0.37-0.48 0.45-0.52

(Continued)

Selected Common Laboratory Values (cont'd)

Test	Conventional Range	SI Range
Hemoglobin	Female: 12-16 g/100 ml	7.4-9.9 mmol/L
	Male: 13-18 g/100 ml	8.1-11.2 mmol/L
Leukocyte count	4300-10,800/cu mm	$4.3\text{-}10.8 \times 10^9$/L
Erythrocyte count	4.2-5.9 million/cu mm	$4.2\text{-}5.9 \times 10^9$/L
Mean corpuscular volume	86-98 m^3 cell	
Mean corpuscular hemoglobin concentration		32%-36%
Creatine kinase	Female: 10-79 U/L	167-1317 nmol sec^{-1}/L
	Male: 17-148 U/L	283-2467 nmol sec^{-1}/L
Creatinine	0.6-1.5 mg/100 ml	53-133 μmol/L
Digoxin	1.2 ± 0.4 mg/ml	1.54 ± 0.5 nmol/L
	1.5 ± 0.4 mg/ml	1.92 ± 0.5 nmol/L
Erythrocyte sedimentation rate	Female: 1-20 mm/hr	1-20 mm/hr
	Male: 1-13 mm/hr	1-13 mm/hr
Folic acid		
Normal	>3.3 ng/ml	>7.3 nmol/L
Borderline	>2.5-3.2 ng/ml	>5.75-7.39 nmol/L
Glucose	Fasting: 70-100 mg/100 ml	3.9-5.6 mmol/L

(Continued)

Selected Common Laboratory Values (cont'd)

Test	Conventional Range	SI Range
Immunoglobulins		
IgG	639-1349 mg/100 ml	6.39-13.49 g/L
IgA	70-312 mg/100 ml	0.7-3.12 g/L
IgM	86-352 mg/100 ml	0.86-3.52 g/L
Iron	50-150 µg/100 ml	9.0-26.9 µmol/L
Lipase	2 units/ml or less	Up to 2 arb. units
Lipids		
Cholesterol	120-220 mg/100 ml	3.10-5.69 mmol/L
Triglycerides	40-150 mg/100 ml	0.4-1.5 g/L
Magnesium	1.5-2.0 mEq/L	0.8-1.3 mmol/L
Partial thrombo-plastin time (activated)	25-38 sec	25-38 sec
Phenytoin	5-20 µg/ml	20-80 µmol/L
Phosphatase (alkaline)	13-39 U/L	217-650 nmol sec^{-1}/L
Phosphorus (inorganic)	3.0-4.5 mg/100 ml	1.0-1.5 mmol/L
Platelet count	150,000-350,000/cu mm	$150-350 \times 10^9$/L
Potassium	3.5-5.0 mEq/L	3.5-5.0 mmol/L
Protein		
Total	6.0-8.4 g/100 ml	60-84 g/L
Albumin	3.5-5.0 g/100 ml	35-50 g/L
Globulin	2.3-3.5 g/100 ml	23-35 g/L
Prothrombin time	Less than 2 sec deviation from control	Less than 2 sec deviation from control

(Continued)

Selected Common Laboratory Values (cont'd)

Test	Conventional Range	SI Range
Reticulocyte count	0.5%-2.5% red cells	0.005-0.025
Salicylate (therapeutic)	20-25 mg/100 ml	1.4-1.8 mmol/L
Sodium	135-145 mEq/L	135-145 mmol/L
Total triiodothyronine (T3)	75-195 ng/100 ml	1.16-3.00 nmol/L
Total thyroxine (T4) by RIA	4-12 µg/100 ml	52-154 nmol/L
Transaminase, SGOT (asparate aminotransferase, AST)	7-27 U/L	117-450 nmol sec^{-1}/L
Transaminase, SGPT (alanine aminotransferase, ALT)	1-21 U/L	17-350 nmol sec^{-1}/L
Urea nitrogen	8-25 mg/100 ml	2.9-8.9 mmol/L
Uric acid	3.0-7.0 mg/100 ml	0.18-0.42 mmol/L
URINE		
Acetone plus acetoacetate	0	0 mg/L
Calcium	<300 hg/d	
Creatinine	15-25 mg/kg body weight/day	0.13-0.22 mmol kg^{-1}/day
Protein	≤150 mg/24 hr	<0.15 g/day
Sugar	0	0 mmol/L
Urobilinogen	Up to 1.0 Ehrlich U	To 1.0 arb. unit

(Continued)

Selected Common Laboratory Values (cont'd)

Test	Conventional Range	SI Range
STOOL		
Fat	Less than 5 g in 24 hr or less than 4% of fat intake in 3 days	<5 g/day
Occult blood	0	0

From Scully RE, editor: Case records of the Massachusetts General Hospital, *N Engl J Med* 314:39-49, January 2, 1986. Reprinted by permission of *The New England Journal of Medicine*.

Appendix E: Guidelines for Home Medical Equipment and Supply Considerations

The most common home medical equipment (HME) for clients in the home setting is listed here. Please consult an HME manual or equipment company representative for any specific coverage or documentation requirements. Medicare has made many changes relating to HME; therefore, consulting the HME representative is very important. Most private insurers have an HME benefit. The specific rules and coverage depend on the insurance program. Physician's orders are needed for all of these items. The term *covered* means that generally, with the appropriate physician documentation and client documented need, this item would be covered for some reimbursement (Marrelli, 1994).

Equipment Coverage by Medicare

Equipment	Indications/Guidelines
Alternating pressure pad and pump (covered)	Client is bedridden and has (or is prone to) decubitus ulcers
Apnea monitor (covered)	Physician documentation needs to be supportive of high-risk history necessitating monitoring for coverage of equipment
Bathtub lifts/seat safety rails (not covered)	Convenience or comfort item, though may be an appropriate safety item
Bedpan (covered)	Bedridden client
Bedside commode (covered)	Impaired ambulation; client confined to room or bed

(Continued)

Equipment Coverage by Medicare (cont'd)

Equipment	Indications/Guidelines
Blood glucose monitoring machine (client dependent)	Usually insulin dependent DM with documentation of poor control history
Cane (covered)	Impaired ambulation condition
Commode (covered)	Client confined to room or bed
Crutches (covered)	Impaired ambulation
Electric hospital bed with rails (covered)	Condition requires frequent change in position, usually cardiac or lung processes and the client can self-operate the controls, otherwise some payers see this as a convenience item for the caregiver (note: overbed table usually not covered; can be rented privately)
Food pumps, enteral feedings (client dependent)	Diagnosis dependent, usually via G-tube or nasogastric tube
Geriatric chair (covered)	Medical need justified by diagnosis in lieu of a wheelchair
High-tech specialty beds including low air-loss beds/mattresses, Clinitrons, etc. (client dependent)	Supportive physician documentation of decubitus ulcer in bed-bound client; refer to HME representative for specific coverage and documentation requirements
Home phototherapy (covered)	Physician documentation supportive of increased bilirubin as documented by venipuncture results
Hospital bed (nonelectric) with rails (covered)	Client usually confined to bed and chair; need for bed must be clearly evident in documentation

(Continued)

Equipment Coverage by Medicare (cont'd)

Equipment	Indications/Guidelines
Hydraulic lift (covered)	Condition requires movement in chair/bedridden client
Infusion pump (covered)	Ordered in conjunction with a course of treatment by physician that is appropriate to client diagnosis
IPPB machine (covered)	Severely impaired respiratory status
Lamb's wool (covered)	Client is usually bed/chair-bound and is prone to decubitus ulcers
Nebulizer (covered)	Severely impaired respiratory status/system
Oxygen therapy equipment (client dependent, if meets diagnostic requirements of blood gas)	Covered conditions include most severe lung disease processes; for ranges of acceptable laboratory values refer to specific HME requirements
Personal emergency response system (not generally covered)	Not seen as therapeutic, although often indicated for clients with history of falls or at risk for falls
Postural drainage board(s) (covered)	Impaired pulmonary status
Quad-cane (covered)	Impaired ambulation condition
Raised toilet seat (not covered)	Seen primarily as a convenience item, though frequently indicated S/P hip surgery
Siderails	Not covered when attached to client's own bed Covered when attached to hospital bed and client qualifies for hospital bed

(Continued)

Equipment Coverage by Medicare (cont'd)

Equipment	Indications/Guidelines
Suction machine (covered)	Based on diagnosis, clinical need, and physician documentation
Telephone alert systems (not generally covered)	Not seen as therapeutic in purpose, though often indicated for elderly clients at risk for falls
TENS unit (covered)	Extensive physician documentation of pain, usually an orthopedic or neurologic diagnosis
Traction equipment (covered)	Orthopedic impairment documented, describing need for equipment by physician
Trapeze (covered)	Bed confinement, need for body position change, or respiratory condition
Walker (covered)	Impaired ambulation condition
Water pressure pads/ mattress (covered)	Client is usually chair/bed-bound and has (or is prone to) decubitus ulcers
Wheelchair (covered)	Bed-bound or chair-bound, specialty wheelchair (note: special sizes or features are based on physician documentation and client condition)

From Marrelli TM: *Handbook of home health standards and documentation guidelines for reimbursement, ed. 2*, St. Louis, 1994, Mosby-Year Book, Inc.

Essential Supplies and Equipment

The following checklist suggests supplies and equipment needed for the home visit.

Home Visit Bag

____   1. Sphygmomanometer
____   2. Stethoscope
      3. Thermometer
         ____ a. Oral
         ____ b. Rectal
____   4. Scissors
____   5. Forceps
____   6. Epinephrine
____   7. TB syringe/needle
____   8. Soap
____   9. Towels
____   10. Apron
____   11. Antiseptic wipes
____   12. Tape measure
____   13. Penlight

Additional Supplies/Equipment for Home Visit

      1. Wound care supplies
         ____ a. 4 x 4
         ____ b. 2 x 2
         ____ c. Kling
         ____ d. Antiseptic solution
         ____ e. Irrigation solution
         ____ f. Other _____
____   2. Asepto syringe
____   3. Intravenous therapy set-up
____   4. Catheter equipment
____   5. Suction catheter
____   6. Irrigation set-up
____   7. Enema
____   8. Ace bandages
____   9. Slings
____   10. Splints
____   11. CPR mask
____   12. Other _____

Stanhope M and Knollmueller RN: *Handbook of community and home health nursing: Tools for assessment, intervention, and education,* St. Louis, 1992, Mosby-Year Book, Inc.

Appendix F: English-Spanish Equivalents of Commonly Used Medical Terms and Phrases

English	Spanish
General phrases	
What is your name?	¿Cómo se llama usted? (¿Cuál es su nombre?)
Where do you work?	¿Dónde trabaja? (Cuál es su profesión o trabajo?) (¿Qué hace usted?)
You will need blood and urine tests.	Usted va a necesitar pruebas de sangre y de orina.
You will be admitted to a hospital.	Usted será ingresado al hospital.
May I help you?	¿Puedo ayudarle?
How are you feeling? Where does it hurt?	¿Cómo se siente? ¿Dónde le duele?
Do you feel better today?	¿Se siente mejor hoy?
Are you sleepy?	¿Tiene usted sueño?
The doctor will examine you now.	El doctor le examinará ahora.
You should remain in bed today.	Usted debe guardar cama hoy.
We want you to get up now.	Queremos que se levante ahora
You may take a bath.	Puede bañarse.
You may take a shower.	Puede tomar una ducha.
Have you noticed any bleeding?	¿Ha notado alguna hemorragia?
Do you still have any numbness?	¿Todavía siente adormecimiento?
Do you have any drug allergies?	¿Es usted alérgico(a) algún médicamento?
I need to change your dressing.	Necesito cambiar su vendaje.
What medications are you taking now?	¿Qué médicamentos está tomando ahora?
Do you take any medications?	¿Toma usted algunas medicinas?

English	Spanish
Do you have a history of	¿Padece
a. heart disease?	a. del corazón?
b. diabetes?	b. de diabetes?
c. epilepsy?	c. de epilepsia?
d. bronchitis?	d. de bronquitis?
e. emphysema?	e. de enfisema?
f. asthma?	f. de asma?
Do you need a sleeping pill?	¿Necesita una pastilla para dormir?
Do you need a laxative?	¿Necesita un laxante/purgante?
Relax. Try to sleep.	Relájese. Trate de dormir.
Please turn on your side.	Favor de ponerse de lado.
Do you have to urinate?	¿Tiene que orinar?
Have you had any sickness from any medicine?	¿Le ha caido mal alguna medicina?
Are you allergic to anything? Medicines, drugs, foods, insect bites?	¿Es usted alérgico(a) a algo? ¿Medicinas, drogas, alimentos, picaduras de insectos?
Do you use contact lenses, dentures? Do you have any loose teeth, removable bridges, or any prosthesis?	¿Usa usted lentes de contacto, dentadura postiza? ¿Tiene dientes flojos, dientes postizos, o cualquier prostesis?

Vocabulary
Anatomy

abdomen	el abdomen
ankle	el tobillo
anus	el ano
appendix	el apéndice
arm	el brazo
back	la espalda
lower back	la cintura
bladder	la vejiga
blood	la sangre
body	el cuerpo
bone	el hueso
bowels	los intestinos, las entrañas
brain	el cerebro
breasts	el pecho, los senos
buttocks	las nalgas, las posaderas, las sentaderas

English	Spanish
calf	la pantorrilla, el chamorro
chest	el pecho
coccyx	la cóccix
collarbone	la clavícula
ear (inner)	el oído
ear (outer)	la oreja
eardrum	el tímpano
ears	las orejas
elbow	el codo
eye	el ojo
face	la cara
fallopian tube	el tubo falopio
finger	el dedo
foot	el pie
genitals	los genitales
hair (of the head)	el pelo, el cabello
hand	la mano
head	la cabeza
heart	el corazón
heart valve	la vávula del corazón
hip	la cadera
hormone	la hormona
intestines	los intestinos
jaw	la quijada
joint	la coyuntura, la articulación
kidney	el riñón
knee	la rodilla
leg	la pierna
ligament	el ligamento
lip	el labio
liver	el hígado
lung	el pulmón
mouth	la boca
muscle	el músculo
neck	el cuello
nerve	el nervio
nose	la nariz
ovary	el ovario
pelvis	la cadera, la pelvis
penis	el pene, el miembro
pulse	el pulso
pupil	la niña del ojo, la pupila

English	Spanish
rib	la costilla
saliva	la saliva
shoulder	el hombro
sinus	el seno
skin	la piel
skin (of the face)	el cutis
skull	el cráneo
spine	el espinazo, la columna vertebral
stomach	el estómago, la panza, la barriga
tendon	el tendón
thigh	el muslo
toe	el dedo del pie
tongue	la lengua
tonsils	las angínas, las amígdalas
tooth, molar	el diente, la muela
trachea	la tráquea
urine	la orina
uterus	el útern, la matriz
vagina	la vagina
vein	la vena
wrist	la muñeca

Common medical problems

abortion	el aborto
abscess	el absceso
appendicitis	la apendicitis
arthritis	la artritis
asthma	el asma
backache	el dolor de espalda
blindness	la ceguera
bronchitis	la bronquitis
bruise	moretón, magulladura
burn (1st, 2nd, or 3rd degree)	la quemadura (de primer, segundo, o tercer grado)
cancer	el cáncer
chickenpox	la varicela
chills	los escalofríos
cold	el catarro, el resfriado
constipation	la constipación
convulsion	la convulsión

English	Spanish
cough	la tos
cramps	los calambres
cut	cortada, cortadura
deafness	la sordera
diabetes	la diabetes
diarrhea	la diarrea
dizziness	el vértigo, el mareo
epilepsy	la epilepsia
fainting spell	el desmayo
fatigue	la fatiga
fever	la fiebre
flu	la influenza, la gripe
food poisoning	el envenamiento por comestibles
fracture	la fractura
gall stone	el cálculo biliar
gastric ulcer	la úlcera gástrica
hallucination	la alucinación
handicap	el impedimento
headache	el dolor de cabeza
heart attack	el ataque al corazón
heartbeat	el latido-el palpito
heart disease	la enfermedad del corazón
heart murmur	el soplo del corazón
hemorrhage	la hemorragia
hemorrhoids	la almorranas
hernia	la hernia
herpes	el herpes
high blood pressure	la presión alta
hives	la urticaria
illness	la enfermedad
immunization	la inmunización
infection	la infección
inflammation	la inflamación
injury	la herida, el daño
itch	la picazón-la comezón
laryngitis	la laringitis
lice	los piojos
malaria	la malaria
malignant	maligno(a)
malnutrition	la mala nutrición
measles	el serampión

English	Spanish
meningitis	la meningitis
menopause	la menopausa
miscarriage	un malparto, un aborto, una perdida
mononucleosis	la mononucleosis infecciosa
multiple sclerosis	la esclerosis multiple
mumps	las paperas
muscular dystrophy	la distrofía muscular
mute	mudo(a)
obese	obeso(a)
obstruction	la obstrucción
overdose	la sobredosis
overweight	el sobrepeso
pain	el dolor
palsy, cerebral	la parálisis cerebral
paralysis	la parálisis
Parkinson's disease	la enfermedad de Parkinson
pneumonia	la pulmonía
poison ivy/oak	la hiedra venenosa
polio	la poliomielitis
rabies	la rabia
rash	la roncha, el salpullido, la erupción
redness	enrojecimiento o inflamación
relapse	la recaída
scar	la cicatriz
shock	el choque
sore	la llaga
spasm	el espasmo
spider bite	la picadura de araña
sprain	la torcedura
stomach ache	el dolor de estómago
sunstroke	la insolación
swelling	la hinchazón
tetanus	el tétano(s)
tonsillitis	la tonsilitis
toothache	el dolor de muela
trauma	el trauma
tuberculosis	la tuberculosis
tumor	el tumor
unconsciousness	la insensibilidad
venereal disease	la enfermedad venérea

English	Spanish
virus	el virus
vomit	el vómito, los vómitos
weakness	la debilidad
welt	roncha, verdugón
whiplash	concusión de la espina cervical, lastimado del cuello

General hospital equipment and supplies

English	Spanish
bandage	la venda
bathtub	la tina
bed	la cama
bedpan	la chata
blanket	la cobi
call bell	el timbre
catheter	el cateter
crutches	las muletas
pillow	la almohada
shower	la ducha
soap	el jabón
stethoscope	el estetoscopio
stretcher	la camilla
syringe	la jeringa
thermometer	el termometro
toilet	el excusado
tongue depressor	el pisalengua
toothbrush	el cepillo de dientes
walker	el apoyador para caminar, el andador
wheelchair	la silla de ruedas

Medications and related supplies

English	Spanish
alcohol	alcohol
amphetamine	anfetamina
antibiotic	antibiótico
application	aplicación
artifical limb	el miembro artificial
aspirin (for children)	aspirina (para niños)
Band-Aid	la curita
barbiturate	barbitúrico
birth control pill	la píldora anticonceptiva
booster shot	la inyección secundaria
brace	el braguero

English	Spanish
calcium	calcio
capsule	cápsula
cocaine	cocaína
codeine	codeína
cold pack	el emplasto frío
compress (hot)	la compresa (caliente)
condom	goma, condón
contact lens	lentes de contacto
contraceptive pills	pastillas anticonceptivas
cotton	algodón
cough syrup	jarabe para la tos
diuretic	diurético
dose	dosis
douche	la ducha, lavado interno
dressing	vendaje
dropper	el gotero
drops	gotas
enema	enema
gauze	gasa
glucose	glucosa
hearing aid	el aparato para la sordera
heroin	heroína
ice	hielo
ice pack	la bolsa de hielo
insulin	insulina
intrauterine device (IUD)	el dispositivio intrauterino
laxative	laxante, purgante. purga
lotion	loción
narcotic	narcótico
needle	aguja
Novocaine	novocaína
ointment	ungüento
pacemaker	el marcapaso
penicillin	penicilina
pill	píldora, pastilla
prosthesis	miembro artificial (prótesis)
sedative	sedante, calmante
sling	el cabestrillo
smelling salts	sales aromáticas
splint	la tablilla
support	el apoyo
suppository	supositorio

English	Spanish
syrup of ipecac	jarabe de ipecacuana
vitamin	vitamina

Medication instructions

English	Spanish
right	derecho(a)
left	izquierdo(a)
tablespoonful	cucharada
teaspoonful	cucharadita
one-half teaspoonful	media cucharadita
BID	dos veces al día
TID	tres veces al día
QID	cuarto veces al día
every hour	cada hora
each day, daily	cada día, diariamente
every other day	cada otro día (cada tercer día)
till gone	hasta terminar (acabar)
Let it dissolve in your mouth.	Que se le disuelva en la boca.
as needed for pain	cuando la necesite para el dolor
symptoms	sintomas
insert	inserte
when you get up in the morning	al levantarse
apply	aplique
one-half hour after meals	una hora antes de comidas
now (stat)	ahora (ahora mismo)
before bedtime	antes de acostarse
before you exercise	antes de hacer ejercicios
chew	mastique
mix	mezcle
dissolved in	disuelto en
Shake well.	Agite bien.
as directed	de acuerdo con las instrucciones
by mouth	por la boca
rub	frote
gargle	haga gargaras
soak	remoje, empape

Tests and procedures

English	Spanish
allergy test	prueba para alergias
analysis	análisis
blood count	recuento (conteo) globular
blood transfusion	la transfusión de sangre
cardiogram	cardiograma

English	Spanish
check-up, medical	reconocimiento (chequeo) médico
culture (throat)	cultivo de la garganta
electrocardiogram	electrocardiograma
electroencephalogram	electroencefalograma
enema	la enema
eye test	examen de la vista (de los ojos)
injection	la inyección
laboratory	laboratorio
massage	el masaje
pregnancy test	prueba de embarazo
specimen	muestra (espécimen)
traction	la tracción
urinalysis	análisis de orina
vaccination	la vacuna
x-rays	radiografias (rayos equis)

Assessment
General

I am _____	Soy _____
I would like to examine you now. Please take off your clothes, except for your underwear (and bra), and put on this gown.	Quisiera examinarlo(a) ahora. Por favor, quítese la ropa menos la ropa interior (y el sostén), y póngase este camisón.
I am going to take your temperature now. Open your mouth.	Le voy a tomar la temperatura ahora. Abra la boca.
I am going to take your blood pressure now.	Le voy a tomar la presión ahora.
Your blood pressure is low.	Su presión es baja.
Your blood pressure is too high.	Su presión es demasiado alta.
Here is a prescription to reduce your blood pressure.	Aquí tiene una receta para bajar la presión de sangre.
You must follow a diet to lose weight.	Debe seguir una dieta para perder peso.
I am going to start an IV.	Le voy a empezar un suero.
Bend your elbow.	Doble el codo.
Make a fist.	Haga un puño.
I am going to give you an injection.	Le voy a poner una inyección.

English	**Spanish**
Breathe normally.	Respire normalmente.
Cough.	Tosa.
Squeeze my hand.	Apriete mi mano.
You have a slight fever.	Ud. tiene un poco de fiebre.
Hold your leg up.	Levante la pierna.
Stand up and walk.	Parese y camine.
Straighten your leg.	Enderece la pierna.
Bend your knee.	Doble la rodilla.
Push/pull.	Empuje/jale.
Up/down.	Arriba/abajo.
In/out.	Adentro/afuera.
Slow/fast.	Despacio/aprisa.
Rest.	Descanse.
Kneel.	Arrodíllese.

Ambulation history

Do you use equipment (canes, crutches, braces)?	¿Usa equipo (bastones, muletas, abrazaderas)?
Do you use a wheelchair?	¿Usa usted una silla de ruedas?
Do you drive a car?	¿Maneja usted un carro?
Can you climb stairs?	¿Puede usted subir las escaleras?

Cardiology

Have you ever had chest pain? Where?	¿Ha tenido alguna vez dolor de pecho? ¿Dónde?
Do you notice any irregularity of heart beat or any palpitations?	¿Nota cualquier latido o palpitación irregular?
Do you get short of breath? When?	¿Tiene falta de aire? ¿Cuándo?
Do you take medicine for your heart? How often?	¿Toma medicina para el corazón? ¿Con qué frecuencia?
Do you know if you have high blood pressure?	¿Sabe usted si tiene la presión alta?
Is there a history of hypertension in your family?	¿Hay historia de hipertensión en su familia?
You have had a heart attack.	Ha tenido un ataque al corazón.

English	Spanish
Be sure to tell us if you have chest pains or if you feel anything unusual.	Debe avisarnos si tiene dolores de pecho o si siente algo anormal.

Diabetes

English	Spanish
You have diabetes.	Usted tiene diabetes.
Your doctor will regulate your dosage.	Su médico le indicará su dosis.

Drug-related problems

English	Spanish
What drugs do you use?	¿Cuáles drogas usa usted?
heroin?	¿heroíns?
cocaine?	¿cocaína?
uppers?	¿estimulantes?
downers?	¿abajos?
barbiturates?	¿diablitos o barbitúricos?
speed?	¿blancas?
Where do you shoot the drugs?	¿Dónde se pone usted las drogas?
Have you ever been through a detoxification program before?	¿Ha participado alguna vez en un programa de desintoxicación?
Have you ever overdosed on drugs?	¿Alguna vez se ha sobredrogado?

Ears, nose, and throat

English	Spanish
Do you have any hearing problems?	¿Tiene Ud. problemas de oír?
Do you use a hearing aid?	¿Usa Ud. un audífono?
Do your ears ring?	¿Siente un tintineo o silbido en los oídos?
Do you have allergies?	¿Tiene alergias?
Do you have a cold?	¿Tiene usted un resfriado/resfrío?
Do you have sore throats frequently?	¿Le duele la garganta con frecuencia?
Have you ever had strep throat?	¿Ha tenido alguna vez "strep" (infección estreptococo de la garganta)?
I want to take a throat culture. Open your mouth. This will not hurt.	Quiero hacer un cultivo de la garganta. Abra la boca. Esto no le va a doler.

English	**Spanish**

Endocrinology

Have you ever had problems with your thyroid?	¿Ha tenido alguna vez problemas con la tiroides?
Have you noted any significant weight gain or loss? What is your usual weight?	¿Ha notado pérdida o aumento de peso? ¿Cuál es su peso usual?
How is your appetite?	¿Qué tal su apetito?
(Women) How old were you when your periods started? How many days between periods? Have you ever been pregnant? How many children do you have?	¿Cuántos años tenía cuando tuvo la primera regla? ¿Cuantos días entre las reglas? ¿Ha estado embarazada? ¿Cuántos hijos tiene?

Gastrointestinal

What foods disagree with you?	¿Qué alimentos le caen mal?
Do you get heartburn?	¿Suele tener ardor en el pecho?
Do you have indigestion often?	¿Tiene indigestión con frecuencia?
Are you going to vomit?	¿Va a vomitar (arrojar)?
Do you have blood in your vomit?	¿Tiene usted vómitos con sangre?

Headaches/head

Do you have headaches?	¿Tiene Ud. dolores de cabeza (jaquecas)?
Do you have migraines?	¿Tiene Ud. migrañas (jaquecas)?
Where is the pain exactly?	¿Dónde le duele, exactamente?
What causes the headaches?	¿Qué la causa los dolores de cabeza?
Are there any changes in your vision?	¿Hay algunos cambios en su vista?

Neurology

Have you ever had a head injury?	¿Ha tenido alguna vez daño a la cabeza?
Have you ever had a sports injury?/motorcycle accident?	¿Ha tenido alguna vez un daño deportivo?/accidente en su motocicleta?
Do you have convulsions?	¿Tiene convulsiones?

English	Spanish
Do you see double?	¿Ve usted doble?
Do you have tingling sensations?	¿Tiene hormigueos?
Do you have numbness in your hands, arms, or feet?	¿Siente entumecidos las manos, los brazos, o los pies?
Have you ever lost consciousness? For how long?	¿Perdió alguna vez el sentido? ¿Por cuánto tiempo?
How frequently does this happen?	¿Con qué frecuencia ocurre esto?
Is this hot or cold?	¿Está frío o caliente esto?
Am I sticking you with the point or the head of the pin?	¿Le estoy pinchando con la cabeza del alfiler?

Obstetrics and gynecoloy

How often do you get your periods?	¿Cada cuándo le viene la regla?
When was your last menstrual period?	¿Cuándo fue su última regla?
When was your last Pap smear?	¿Cuándo fue su última prueba de Pap?
Would you like information on birth control methods?	¿Quiere usted información sobre los métodos del control de la natalidad? (los métodos anticonceptivos)?
Do you have an IUD in place?	¿Le han puesto un aparato intrauterino?

Ophthalmology

Have you had pain in your eyes?	¿Ha tenido dolor en los ojos?
Do you wear glasses?	¿Usa usted anteojos/gafas/lentes/espejuelos?
Were you exposed to anything that could have injured your eye?	¿Fue expuesto a cualquier cosa que pudiera haberle dañado el ojo?
Do your eyes water much?	¿Le lagrimean mucho los ojos?
I am going to put drops in your eyes in order to examine them. This medicine may burn at first.	Le voy a poner gotas en los ojos para examinarlos. Esta medicina puede arderle al principio.

English	**Spanish**

Orthopedics

You have broken (a bone).	Usted se ha quebrado/roto (un hueso).
You have dislocated (a joint).	Usted se ha dislocado (una coyuntura).
You have pulled (a muscle).	Usted se ha distendido (un músculo).
You have sprained (a muscle)/(a ligament).	Usted se ha torcido (un músculo)/(un ligamento).
You will need a cast.	Necesita un yeso.
Do you feel pain when you stand?	¿Siente dolor a pararse?
Do you feel pain when you bend?	¿Siente dolor al doblarse?
We need to take some x-rays.	Necesitamos tomarle unos rayos X.
You must wear a sling whenever you are out of bed.	Usted debe llevar un cabestrillo cuando no este en la cama.

Pain

What were you doing when the pain started?	¿Qué hacía usted cuando le comenzó el dolor?
Where is the pain?	¿Dónde está el dolor?
How severe is the pain? Mild, moderate, sharp, or severe?	¿Qué tan fuerte es el dolor? ¿Ligero, moderado, agudo, severo?
Have you ever had this pain before?	¿Ha tenido este dolor antes? (¿Ha sido siempre así?)
Does it hurt when I press here? How did the accident happen?	¿Le duele cuando le aprieto aquí? ¿Cómo sucedió el accidente?
How did this happen? How long ago?	¿Cómo sucedió esto? ¿Cuánto tiempo hace?

Pulmonary/respiratory

Do you smoke? How many packs a day?	¿Fuma usted? ¿Cuántos paquentes al día?
How long have you been coughing?	¿Desde cúando tiene tos?
Does it hurt when you cough?	¿Le duele cuando tose?

English	Spanish
Do you cough up phlegm?	¿Al toser, escupe usted flema(s)?
Do you cough up blood?	¿Al toser, arroja usted sangre?
Do you wheeze?	¿Le silba a usted el pecho?
Have you ever had asthma?	¿Ha tenido asma alguna vez?
Have you ever had	¿Ha tenido alguna vez
tuberculosis?	tuberculosis?
pneumonia?	pulmonía?
emphysema?	enfisema?
bronchitis?	bronquitis?
Breathe deeply.	Aspire profundamente. (Respire profundo.)

Sexually transmitted diseases

Do you have urethral discharge?	¿Tiene descarga de la uretra?
Do you have burning with urination?	¿Tiene ardor al orinar?
Do you have a vaginal discharge?	¿Tiene descargas vaginales?
Do you have abdominal pain?	¿Tiene dolor en el abdomen?
When did you last have intercourse?	¿Cuándo fue la última vez que tuvo relaciones sexuales?

Unconscious patient

What happened to him/her?	¿Que le pasó? (Que le sucedió?)
Has he vomited?	¿Ha vomitado?
Is she pregnant?	¿Está embarazada?

Patient Instructions
General

Roll over and sit up over the edge of the bed.	Voltéese y siétese sobre el borde de la cama.
Stand up slowly. Put weight only on your right/left foot.	Párese despacio. Ponga peso sólo en la pierna derecha/izquierda.
Lift your head up.	Levante la cabeza.
Take a step to the side.	Dé un paso al lado.
Turn to your left/right.	Doble a la izquierda/derecha.

English	**Spanish**

Drugs

English	Spanish
I want you to take your medicine.	Quiero que tome su medicina.
Let it dissolve in your mouth.	Que se le disuelva en la boca.
Apply _____ to the affected part.	Aplique _____ en la parte afectada.
Cool in the refrigerator.	Enfrie en el refrigerador.
Here is some medication for _____. Take _____ tablets every _____ hours as needed.	Aquí tiene la medicina para _____. Tome _____ tabletas cada _____ horas según la necesite.
These pills are vitamins.	Estas pastillas son vitaminas.
These pills are for pain.	Estas pastillas son para dolor.
Take _____ of these pills each day.	Tome ___ de estas pastillas cada día.
Here is enough medicine for _____ days.	Aquí tiene suficiente medicina para _____ días.
Take one of these pills every _____ hours.	Tome una de estas pastillas cada _____ horas.
Take one pill daily for _____ days.	Tome una pastilla por _____ días.
But no more than _____ a day maximurn.	Pero no más de _____ en total cada día.
Fill the medicine dropper to this line and mix with a glass of water, juice, or milk.	Llene el gotero hasta esta línea y mezcle con un vaso de agua, jugo, o leche.
It is important for you to eat/drink liquids.	Es importante que usted coma/beba o tome líquidos.

From Lister S, Wilber CJ: *Medical Spanish: The instant survival guide*, London, 1983, Butterworth.

Appendix G: Guide to Supplemental and Educational Resources

Directory of Resources

Accent on Information: (309) 378-2961

Agency for Health Care Policy and Research (AHCPR): 1-800-358-9295. (AHCPR has a congressional mandate for developing clinical practice guidelines. Free copies of released guidelines are available.)

AIDS Adult and Pediatric Clinical Trials Information Services: 1-800-874-2572 or 1-800-TRIALS-A

AIDS Hotline, National: 1-800-342-2437 or 1-800-342-AIDS

AIDS Hotline, National, Spanish: 1-800-344-7432

AIDS Medical Foundation: (212) 206-0670

AIDS, National Information Clearinghouse, CDC: 1-800-458-5231

Alliance for Aging Research: (202) 293-2856

Alzheimer's Disease and Other Related Disorders Association: 1-800-621-0379 or (312) 853-3060

Alzheimer's Disease Educational and Referral Center (NIH, National Institute on Aging): 1-800-438-4380

American Association of Kidney Patients: (813) 254-2558

American Association of Retired Persons (AARP): (202) 872-4700

American Brain Tumor Association: 1-800-886-2282 or (312) 286-5571

American Cancer Society: 1-800-ACS-2345

American Cancer Society: 1-800-395-LOOK. ("Look Good . . . Feel Better" program for women undergoing chemotherapy or radiation)

American Cleft Palate Association: (412) 681-9620

American Council of the Blind: 1-800-424-8666 or (202) 833-1251

American Diabetes Association: 1-800-232-6366 or (212) 683-7444

American Dietetic Association: (313) 280-5012

American Fertility Association: (205) 251-9764

American Federation of Home Health Agencies: (301) 588-1454

American Foundation for the Blind: 1-800-232-5463

American Foundation for Urologic Disease: 1-800-828-7866

American Heart Association: 1-800-242-8721 or (214) 750-5300

American Lung Association: 1-800-232-5861

American Hospital Association: (312) 280-6000

American Nurses Association: (202) 554-4444

American Occupational Therapy Association: 1-800-426-2547

American Physical Therapy Association: (703) 684-2782

American Red Cross: (202) 737-8300; consult telephone directory for local office

American Society on Aging: (415) 543-2617

American Speech-Language-Hearing Association: 1-800-638-8255

Arthritis Foundation: (404) 872-7100

Association of Nurses in AIDS Care: (215) 321-2371

Association for Retarded Citizens (ARC) of the United States: (817) 640-0204

Breast Cancer Patient Resource: 1-800-221-2141. (The Y-Me Hotline for women who want to talk with other women with breast cancer)

Cancer Federation, Inc.: 1-800-982-3270

Cancer Care, Inc.: (212) 221-3300

Cancer Information Service (CIS): 1-800-4-CANCER

Canadian Nurses Association, 50 The Driveway, Ottawa, Ontario K2P1E2

CDC National AIDS Clearinghouse: 1-800-458-5231

Children with AIDS Project of America: 1-800-866-2437

Continence Restored, Inc.: (212) 879-3131

Council of Community Health Services, National League for Nursing: (212) 582-1022 or (301) 881-9130

Cystic Fibrosis Foundation: 1-800-FIGHT-CF or (301) 881-9130

Elder Care Locator Services: 1-800-677-1116

Environmental Protection Agency: Send for the following free brochures: (1) *Disposal Tips for Home Health Care; Educating Your Patients;* (2) *Disposal Tips for Home Health Care:* and (3) *Handle with Care, How to Throw Out Used Insulin Syringes and Lancets at Home, a Booklet for Young People with Diabetes and Their Families.*

FDA's "Product Problem Reporting Program": 1-800-638-6725

Foundation for Hospice and Home Care: (202) 547-7424

Gray Panthers: (212) 382-3300

Head and Neck Cancer Information Service: 1-800-368-1422

Help for Incontinent People (HIP): 1-800-252-3337 or 1-800-BLADDER

Hospice Association of America: (202) 546-4759

Hospice Nurses Association, P.O. Box 8166, Van Nuys, CA 91409

International Center for Social Gerontology: (202) 479-2642

La Leche League: (312) 455-7730

Leukemia Society of America, Inc.: 1-800-955-4LSA or (212) 573-8484

Make-A-Wish Foundation of America: 1-800-722-9474 or (602) 240-6060

March of Dimes Birth Defects Foundation: (914) 428-7100

Meals on Wheels: consult telephone directory for local office

Medic Alert Foundation International: 1-800-344-3226 or (209) 668-3333

Muscular Dystrophy Association: (212) 586-0808

National Association for Home Care (NAHC): (202) 547-7424

National Association for the Deaf: (301) 587-1788

National Association of Area Agencies on Aging: (202) 484-7520

National Association of Physically Handicapped, Inc.: (614) 852-1664

National Brain Tumor Foundation: 1-800-934-CURE or (415) 296-0404

National Cancer Institute: (301) 496-5583

National Coalition for Cancer Research: (202) 544-1880

National Council of Senior Citizens: (202) 347-8800

National Council on Patient Information and Education: (202) 347-6711

National Council on the Aging: (202) 479-1200

National Easter Seal Society: (312) 243-8400

National Foundation for Ileitis and Colitis: 1-800-343-3637

National Hemophiliac Foundation: (212) 431-8541

National Hospice Organization: 1-800-658-8898 or (703) 243-5900

National Information Center on Deafness: (202) 651-5109

National Institute on Aging: (301) 496-1752

National Institute of Arthritis, Diabetes, and Digestive and Kidney Diseases: (301) 496-7495 or (301) 496-9707

National Institute of Mental Health: (301) 443-2403

National Kidney and Urologic Diseases Information Clearinghouse: (301) 468-6345

National Kidney Foundation: 1-800-622-9010 or (212) 889-2210

National Library of Congress Referral Center: (202) 287-5670. (This is a free referral service that can help the professional nurse locate information or identify needed services.)

National Lymphedema Network: 1-800-541-3259

National Multiple Sclerosis Society: (212) 986-3240

National Rehabilitation Association: (703) 836-0850

National Spinal Cord Injury Association: (617) 964-0521

Oncology Nursing Society: (412) 921-7373

People with AIDS Coalition: 1-800-828-3280

Prostate Cancer Support Group (Us Too): 1-800-82-US-TOO or 1 -800-828-7866

Skin Cancer Foundation: (212) 725-5176

Spina Bifida Association of America (SBAA): (301) 770-SBAA

United Cerebral Palsy Association: (212) 481-6316

United Ostomy Association: (714) 660-8624 or (213) 413-5510 or 1-800-826-0826

United Way: consult telephone directory for local office

Visiting Nurse Association of America: 1-800-426-2547

Y-Me National Organization for Breast Cancer Information and Support: (708) 799-8338

Adapted from Marrelli TM: *Handbook of home health standards and documentation guidelines for reimbursement, ed. 2*, St. Louis, 1994, Mosby-Year Book, Inc.

Clinical Newsletters and Journals

The American Journal of Hospice and Palliative Care, 470 Boston Post Road, Weston, MA 02193, 1-800-869-2700.

Caring magazine is published monthly by the National Association for Home Care. Inquiries for subscription and/or membership can be directed to The National Association for Home Care at 519 C Street, NE, Washington, DC 20002-5809.

Home Care Nurse News is a monthly newsletter published by Tina M. Marrelli, Suite 159, 3 Church Circle, Annapolis, MD 21401, 1-800-993-NEWS (6397).

Home Health Care Nurse is published bimonthly by J.B. Lippincott Company, 12107 Insurance Way, Hagerstown, MD 21740.

Home Health Care Pharmacy and Therapeutics Update is a monthly newsletter that addresses updates on new drugs, reviews therapeutic issues, and has "Drug Information" and "Hospice Happenings" columns. This newsletter, which answers questions submitted by HHA and hospice staff, is $20 for an annual subscription. Written inquiries should be directed to Sinai Home Care-Hospice Program, Attn: Dr. Lynn McPherson, 21 Crossroad Drive, Suite 450, Owings Mills, MD 21117; or the newsletter can be ordered by calling (410) 356-9112.

Home Health Focus is a monthly newsletter published by Mosby-Year Book, Inc., 11830 Westline Industrial Drive, St. Louis, MO 63146, 1-800-453-4351. The editor-in-chief is Karen Martin, RN, MSN, FAAN.

The Hospice Journal is published by The Haworth Press, Inc., 10 Alice Street, Bingingham, NY 13904, 1-800-342-9678.

Journal of Home Health Care Practice is published quarterly by Aspen Publishers, Inc., 7201 McKinney Circle, Frederick, MD 21781, 1-800-638-8437.

Adapted from Marrelli TM: *Handbook of home health standards and documentation guidelines for reimbursement, ed. 2*, St. Louis, 1994, Mosby-Year Book, Inc.

References

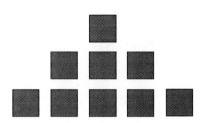

A Statement on the Scope of Home Health Nursing Practice, Washington, DC, 1992, American Nurses Association.

American Diabetes Association: Nutritional recommendations for individuals with diabetes mellitus: 1986, *Diabetes Care* 10, 1987, p. 126.

American Hospital Association: *A patient's bill of rights,* Chicago, 1992, The Association.

American Pain Society: *Principles of analgesic use in the treatment of acute pain and chronic cancer pain, ed. 2,* Skokie, Ill., 1989, The Society.

Barker E: *Neuroscience Nursing,* St. Louis, 1994, Mosby-Year Book, Inc.

Barnett JH, Mohr JP, Stein BM, and Yatsu FM: *Stroke: Pathophysiology, diagnosis, and management,* New York, 1986, Churchill Livingstone, Inc.

Bauvette-Risey J: Nervous System. In Burggraf V and Stanley M, eds.: *Nursing the elderly: A care plan approach*, Philadelphia, 1989, JB Lippincott Co.

Beare PG and Myers JL: *Principles and practice of adult health nursing, ed. 2,* St. Louis, 1994, Mosby-Year Book, Inc.

Bergenstal R: Acute and chronic complications of diabetes, *Caring* 3(11), November, 1988. Reprinted by permission of the National Association for Home Care.

Bobak IM and Jensen MD: *Maternity and gynecologic care: The nurse and the family, ed. 5*, St. Louis, 1993, Mosby-Year Book, Inc.

Bobak IM, Jensen MD, and Lowdermilk DL: *Maternity nursing, ed. 4*, St. Louis, 1995, Mosby-Year Book, Inc.

Bronstein KS, Popovich JM, Stewart-Amidei C: *Promoting stroke recovery: A research-based approach for nurses,* St. Louis, 1991, Mosby-Year Book, Inc.

Collopy B, Dubler N, and Zuckerman C: The ethics of home care: Autonomy and accommodation, *The Hastings Center Report* 20(2) (suppl):3, 1990

Creasia JL and Parker B: *Conceptual foundations of professional nursing practice*, St. Louis, 1991, Mosby-Year Book, Inc.

Dahl JL, Joranson DE, Engber D, and Dosch J: The cancer pain problem: Wisconsin's response, *J Pain Symp Manag* 3(1):52-58, 1988.

Day JA, Mason RR, and Chesrown SE: Effects of massage on serum level of beta-endorphin and beta-lipotropin in health adults, *Phys Ther* 67(6), 926-930, 1987.

Detlefs DR and Meyers RJ: *1992 Guide to social security and Medicare,* Baltimore, 1991, Department of Health and Human Services.

Dettenmeier PA: *Pulmonary nursing care,* St. Louis, 1992, Mosby-Year Book, Inc.

Dickason EJ, Schultz MO, and Silverman BL: *Maternal and infant nursing care, ed. 2,* St. Louis, 1994, Mosby-Year Book, Inc.

Ebersole P and Hess P: *Toward healthy aging: Human needs and nursing response, ed. 4,* St. Louis, 1994, Mosby-Year Book, Inc.

Escher JE, O'Dell C, and Gambert SR: Typical geriatric accidents and how to prevent them, *Geriatric* 44:57, 1989.

Folcik MA, Carini-Garcia G, and Birmingham JJ: *Traction: Assessment and management,* St. Louis, 1994, Mosby-Year Book, Inc.

Giger JN and Davidhizar RE: *Transcultural nursing, ed. 2,* St. Louis, 1995, Mosby-Year Book, Inc. (in press).

Goodner B: *The nurse's survival guide, ed. 2,* El Paso, Tex., 1993, Skidmore-Roth Publishing, Inc.

Health Care Financing Administration Fact Sheets, Department of Health and Human Services, November 1991.

Health Care Financing Administration: *Federal Register* 54:(155) :33354-33373, Washington, DC, 1989, Department of Health and Human Services.

Hogstel MO: *Clinical manual of gerontological nursing,* St. Louis, 1992, Mosby-Year Book, Inc.

Hughes A, Marlin J, and Franks P: *AIDS home care and hospice manual,* VNA of San Francisco, 1987, AIDS Home Care and Hospice Program.

Jaffe MS and Skidmore-Roth L: *Home health nursing care plans, ed. 2,* St. Louis, 1993, Mosby-Year Book, Inc.

Kaada B and Torsteinbo O: Increases of plasma beta-endorphins in connective tissue massage, *Gen Pharmacol* 20(4), 487-489, 1989.

Katz S, et al.: Studies of illness in the aged, *JAMA* 185, September 21, 1963.

LaRocca JC: *Handbook of home care IV therapy,* St. Louis, 1994, Mosby-Year Book, Inc.

Lister S and Wilber CJ: *Medical Spanish: The instant survival guide*, London, 1983, Butterworth.

Long BC, Phipps WJ, and Cassmeyer VL: *Medical-surgical nursing: A nursing process approach, ed. 3,* St. Louis, 1993, Mosby-Year Book, Inc.

Marrelli TM: *Handbook of home health standards and documentation guidelines for reimbursement, ed. 2,* St. Louis, 1994, Mosby-Year Book, Inc.

Martinson I and Widmer J, eds: *Home health care nursing,* Philadelphia, 1989, WB Saunders Co.

McCaffery M and Beebe A: *Pain: Clinical manual for nursing practice*, St. Louis, 1989, C.V. Mosby Company.

McCance KL and Huether SE: *Pathophysiology: The biological basis for disease in adults and children, ed. 2,* St. Louis, 1994, Mosby-Year Book, Inc.

Mosby's medical, nursing, and allied health dictionary, ed. 4, St. Louis, 1994, Mosby-Year Book, Inc.

Mourad L: *Orthopedic disorders*, St. Louis, 1990, Mosby-Year Book, Inc.

Mumma CM, ed: *Rehabilitation nursing concepts and practice: A core curriculum, ed. 2*, Skokie, Ill., 1987, Rehabilitation Nursing Foundation.

National Stroke Association: *The road ahead: A stroke recovery guide,* Englewood, Colo., 1989, The Association.

Perry AG and Potter PA: *Clinical nursing skills and techniques, ed. 3,* St. Louis, 1994, Mosby-Year Book, Inc.

Portenoy RK and Hagen NA: Breakthrough pain: Definition and management, *Oncology,* 3(suppl 8), 25-29, 1989.

Potter PA and Perry AG: *Fundamentals of nursing: Concepts, process, and practice, ed. 3,* St. Louis, 1993, Mosby-Year Book, Inc.

Redman BK: *The Process of Patient Education, ed, 7.* St. Louis, 1993, Mosby-Year Book, Inc.

Rice R: *Home health nursing practice,* St. Louis, 1992, Mosby-Year Book, Inc.

Scully RE, editor: Case records of the Massachusetts General Hospital, *N Engl J Med* 314: 39-49, January 2, 1986.

Stanhope M and Knollmueller RN: *Handbook of community and home health nursing: Tools for assessment, intervention, and education,* St. Louis, 1992, Mosby-Year Book, Inc.

Stanhope M and Lancaster J: *Community health nursing: process and practice for promoting health, ed. 3,* St. Louis, 1992, Mosby-Year Book, Inc.

Stulginsky MM: Nurses' home health experience. Part I: The practice setting, *Nursing and Health Care,* 14: 8, 403-407, 1993.

Tideiksaar R: New York, 1983, Ritter Department of Geriatrics and Adult Development, The Mount Sinai Medical Center.

Turner J, McDonald G, and Larter N: *Handbook of pediatric and adult respiratory home care,* St. Louis, 1994, Mosby-Year Book, Inc.

Twardon C, Gartner M, and Cherry C: A competency achievement orientation program: Professional development of the home health nurse, *Journal of Nursing Administration* 23:7/8, 20-25, 1993.

Watt-Watson JH and Donovan MI: *Pain management: A nursing perspective,* St. Louis, 1992, Mosby-Year Book, Inc.

Weber F: Tips on implementing the patient self-determination act, *Nursing and Health Care* 1993:2, 86-92.

Weilitz PA: *Pocket guide to respiratory care,* St. Louis, 1991, Mosby-Year Book, Inc.

Wilson SF and Thompson JM: *Respiratory disorders,* St. Louis, 1990, Mosby-Year Book, Inc.

Winthrop E: *Client teaching tips*, in *Mosby's Patient Teaching Guides*, St. Louis, 1995, Mosby-Year Book, Inc.

Index

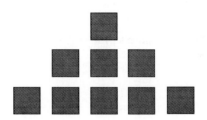

A